# *Live Better* Ayurveda

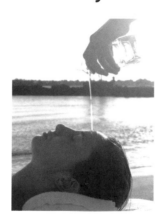

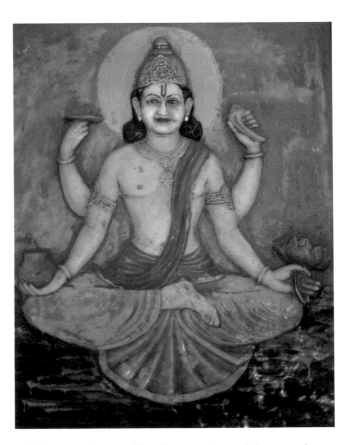

Dhanwantari - The Originator of Ayurveda

# Live Better Ayurveda

remedies and inspirations for well-being

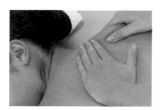

# Dr Donn Brennan

DUNCAN BAIRD PUBLISHERS

LONDON

# Live Better: Ayurveda

Dr Donn Brennan

First published in the United Kingdom
and Ireland in 2006 by
Duncan Baird Publishers Ltd
Sixth Floor
Castle House
75–76 Wells Street
London W1T 3QH

Conceived, created and designed by
Duncan Baird Publishers Ltd
Copyright © Duncan Baird Publishers 2006
Text copyright © Dr Donn Brennan 2006
Commissioned photography copyright © Duncan Baird
Publishers 2006
For copyright of agency photographs see p.128, which is to
be regarded as an extension of this copyright.

Managing Designer: Manisha Patel
Designer: Justin Ford
Managing Editor: Grace Cheetham
Editor: Kirsty Seymour-Ure
Picture Research: Susannah Stone

British Library Cataloguing-in-Publication Data:
A CIP record for this book is available from the
British Library.

ISBN: 978-1-84483-291-0

10 9 8 7 6 5 4 3 2

Typeset in Filosofia and Son Kern
Colour reproduction by Scanhouse, Malaysia
Printed by Imago, Malaysia

**Publisher's note**

Before following any advice or practice suggested in
this book, it is recommended that you consult your
doctor as to its suitability, especially if you suffer
from any health problems or special conditions.
The publishers, author and photographers cannot
accept any responsibility for any injuries or damage
incurred as a result of following the exercises in this
book, or of using any of the therapeutic techniques
described or mentioned here.

The abbreviations BCE and CE are used throughout
this book, meaning respectively Before the
Common Era (equivalent to BC) and Common Era
(equivalent to AD).

# contents

# Introduction

The word *Ayurveda* means "knowledge of life". And the purpose of Ayurveda? To add years to your life and life to your years.

Ayurveda is the traditional health system that developed in India thousands of years ago. Concerned as it is with a deep knowledge of the dynamics structuring the whole of life, Ayurveda is now undergoing a revival across the globe, empowering people to heal themselves.

Health is natural, and is a state of balance. To live your most balanced state of vitality and joy is easy, because being balanced requires least energy. It requires effort to create any imbalance in mind-body: creating disease – a "lack of ease" – uses a great deal of energy and resources. Just a little energy and time spent absorbing and using Ayurveda will empower you to regain, and maintain, your natural state of health.

Ayurveda provides maintenance for the mind and body. In the same way that failing to service your car and driving it roughly leads to problems, so failing to understand your mind-body and not treating it with due regard creates increasing imbalance, leading to disease.

The knowledge of Ayurveda is vital in illness. Pain is a signal of distress and imbalance, telling us that something is wrong. It becomes terrible only if we do not understand what it is telling us about how to re-create balance. Ayurveda enables you to understand what your pain is about and what you can do to heal.

Chapter One of this book describes Ayurveda's history and perspective. Chapter Two explains the three Ayurvedic principles that structure and support life. The third chapter informs on how to enjoy health in body, mind and spirit by maintaining these principles in balance in ourselves, and how to use them to heal ourselves when ill. And the Ayurvedic cycles and how they affect our lives are explored in Chapter Four.

I invite you to read on and learn how to create balance and health by discovering what is right for you. Understand the routine, recreation, exercise, food and lifestyle that suits you best — and regain your natural state of living in joy, love, happiness, harmony and health.

# ayurveda for today

Ayurveda, the world's most ancient known tradition of health, is now undergoing a vigorous revival not only in the place of its birth, India, but also throughout the world because it is capable of meeting the needs of our time. The two Sanskrit words *ayus* and *veda* together mean "knowledge of life".

Ayurveda is a complete medical system that has evolved over time, integrating centuries of wisdom derived from experience. Holistic medicine at its best, Ayurveda describes all aspects of health – physical, mental, spiritual, social, environmental – all aspects of the relationship between the individual and the universe, and how all these aspects are handled so as to generate health. The importance of a person's lifestyle and dietary habits and their appropriate variation in different seasons are understood. Treatment and management of diseases are described; though it is an ancient system, the benefits of many Ayurvedic herbals are validated by modern science.

While Ayurveda is a complete and complex system, its fundamental principles are simple and practical to use. It is easy to integrate them into your life and create better health for yourself and your loved ones. As much about staying healthy as curing ill-health, Ayurveda enables you to recognize your unique nature and to live to your full potential.

# THE HISTORY OF AYURVEDA

Although the origins of Ayurveda are shrouded in the mists of time, it seems that more than 2,500 years ago the principles upon which our lives are based, together with an understanding of how – today, as then – we can be healthy, were being passed down from father to son in families devoted to healing.

In 3000BCE some of the greatest cities on earth were in the Indus Valley in what is now Pakistan and western India, and this may have been where Ayurveda began. The Rig-Veda, the first of the four Hindu scriptures and the world's oldest written document, includes descriptions of surgery, prosthesis and the use of 67 herbs. By 1200BCE there were 100 diseases and eight medical specialities enumerated. The Vedic literature developed with many different branches of knowledge; Ayurveda, the Vedic science of healing, is reckoned by historians to have been formulated as we now know it c.500BCE.

In the 3rd century BCE most of India was ruled over by the Buddhist king Ashoka. Under his patronage there were gardens of medicinal herbs in towns and Ayurvedic hospitals dispensed free medicines. Ashoka supported Ayurveda's spread through eastern Asia, catalyzing the development of Chinese medicine. Around the same time, the Greek physician Hippocrates was developing similar ideas. Ayurvedic texts in translation went on to stimulate the development of Arabic medicine, which subsequently influenced medicine in Europe.

The teaching and practice of Ayurveda were suppressed in India from around the 12th century while the subcontinent was under Muslim and then British rule. Only in the early 1900s did Ayurveda begin to recover. In India today there are more than 300,000 Ayurvedic practitioners, or *vaidyas*, treating the 60 percent of Indians who use Ayurveda as their primary health-care system. The Indian government is beginning seriously to promote this indigenous medical system.

This is partly due to growing international interest. Ayurvedic courses and practitioners' associations are springing up throughout the West and in Japan, indicative of the new status of this ancient system.

# OTHER VEDIC APPROACHES

There are six schools of Vedic philosophy that inform and bring a coherent logic to Ayurveda. These and all other Vedic sciences share the same perspective: you are a spiritual person manifesting a physical structure and not a physical body projecting a spirit. They describe the expression of your life from an inner source of pure consciousness and use this insight to help you generate a fulfilled life using the appropriate Vedic knowledge.

Stapathya-veda is the science of Vedic architecture – the building of houses and town planning according to natural principles. Living in such buildings is thought to enhance health. Ghandharva-veda, the Vedic knowledge of music, describes different rhythms and music for different times. Listening to music associated with a given time regulates your body's rhythms appropriately for that time and so improves health. Jyotish, or Vedic astrology, deals with your relationship with the universe. It offers prescriptions for gems and *yagyas*, formulas performed by Vedic *pandits*, or priests.

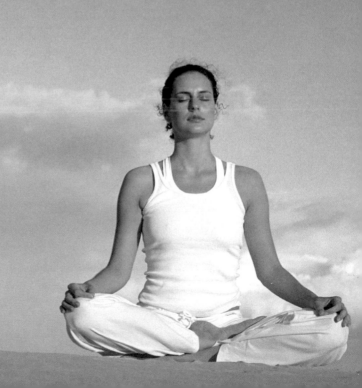

# WHAT IS AYURVEDA?

Variety is the spice of life. Some plants like the sun; others like the shade. Some grow in sandy soil, while others prefer damp, boggy earth. The polar bear thrives in the Arctic, lizards in the desert.

Similarly, human beings have different natures and needs. Yet differences, while giving variety and joy to life, also mean that what is good for one person may not suit another. To be healthy, we each need to know our own unique nature, and the things that are good (and bad) for us – otherwise we resemble car owners who don't know whether to use petrol or diesel, what type of oil is right, or when to service the car.

A complete system of health care has to understand us, and the universe around us, and the connection between ourselves and the universe. From all the possibilities available, it must be able to show us how to choose what we need, and how to avoid what we don't need, in order to be healthy and happy. Ayurveda is a practical system that helps us to understand not only ourselves, but also our connection with the world. It can teach us how to get in touch with ourselves at a very deep level, how to love ourselves profoundly and how to care for our physical body, as well as how to love and respect plants, animals and the whole of nature that surrounds us and from which we can draw health.

A key tool in Ayurveda is the classification of three fundamental principles, known as *vata*, *pitta* and *kapha*. These principles determine the individual qualities of every person and how they relate to their surroundings. From them, you can select the right elements to create balance in your life. As modern science has shown, there are patterns in nature. events do not happen in a completely random way. Once such patterns and principles are understood, we can make huge progress in harnessing the connections between ourselves and the universe. This doesn't just mean discovering electricity, or the secrets of flight, or any of the many other wonderful transformations of the past. It also means discovering the blueprint for perfect health in our own lives – in many ways, the most exciting transformation of all.

# KNOWLEDGE OF LIFE

To enjoy life to the full, you must be fully healthy. The "knowledge of life" contained in Ayurveda for millennia empowers you to take control of your health.

As we will see, everything in life and in the universe has qualities. Food is hot or cold, oily or dry, heavy or light. The weather may be damp or dry. The company you keep – is it cheerful or dull? The qualities of everything around you will interact with your own unique qualities either to improve or to disrupt your health.

Perhaps you are a warm, compassionate person? Steady? Quick? Ayurveda describes you in terms of such qualities, and such a description includes body, mind, emotions, and the person as a whole.

Opposite qualities balance each other: and according to Ayurveda the secret of health is to be balanced. If you are feeling cold, you naturally choose heat. If you are full after overeating, you eat lightly at your next meal. By understanding your own qualities and how to keep them in balance, you can choose how to be healthier.

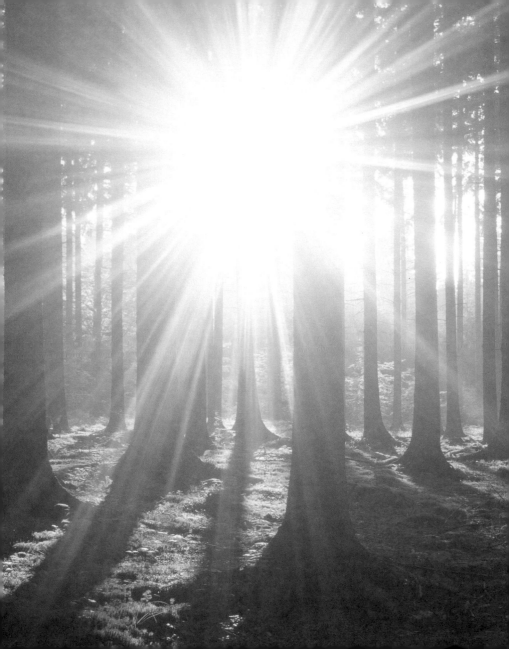

They live in wisdom who see themselves in all
and all in them.

BHAGAVAD GITA

(6TH CENTURY BCE)


No man is an Island, entire of itself; every man is a
piece of the Continent, a part of the main.

JOHN DONNE

(1572–1631)

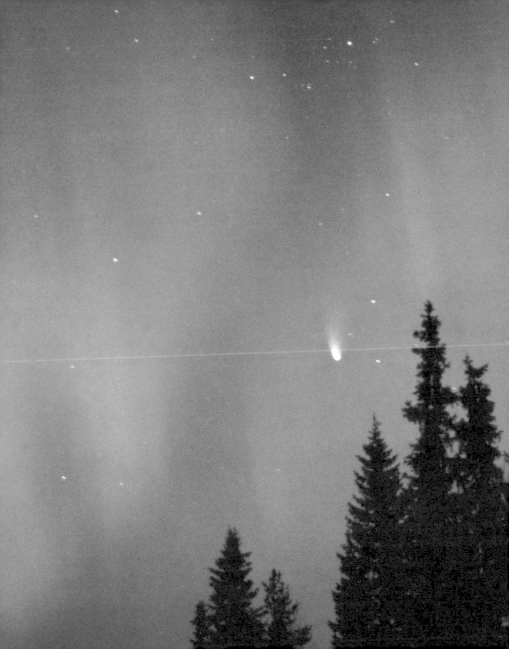

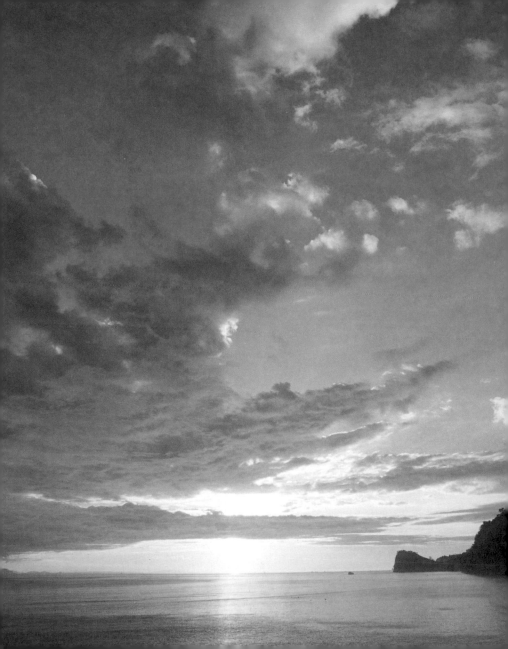

# THE FIVE ELEMENTS

All experiences occur to us through five senses. You hear your own thoughts. Using touch internally you feel emotion. Your inner sight visualizes the ocean hundreds of miles away. "Sweet" joy and "bitter" grief you experience via the senses of taste and smell.

Ayurveda explains how you project five subtle elements through your five senses. Through the sense of hearing the element of space is generated. Through touch the air element arises. The fire element is projected by the sense of sight. Water and earth elements arise from the senses of taste and smell respectively.

These are the five basic elements in life, and they form the building blocks of the universe. In all living beings these five elements are dynamic and work together to structure life. Space and air elements work together as *vata*. Fire and water elements become *pitta*. Water and earth elements make up *kapha*. This is how *vata*, *pitta* and *kapha* originate within you, to become the qualities that define you, as explained in Chapter Two.

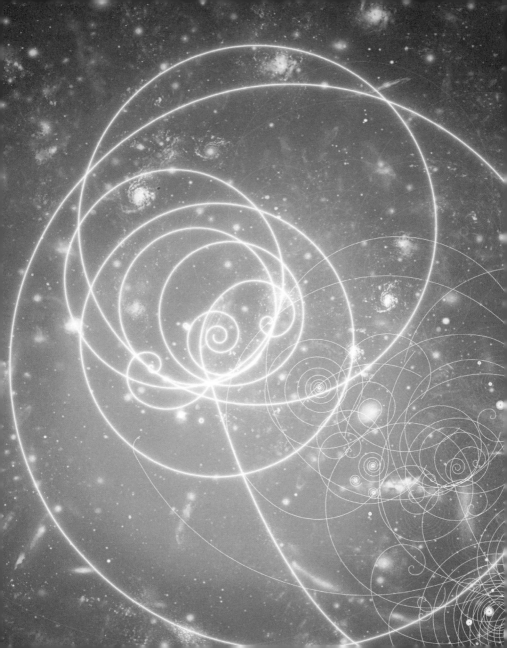

# MODERN SCIENCE AND VEDIC SCIENCE

While Ayurveda is an age-old discipline, its viewpoint is remarkably compatible with 21st-century scientific thinking. Physics no longer sees the universe as purely physical, but rather as energy: the universe is made up of atoms, and atoms are made up of subatomic particles that are actually little bundles of energy. This energy is therefore at the core of all physical reality and makes up the particles from which all matter is formed.

Quantum mechanics describes a certain number of elementary particles, which are related to one another by forces or fields of energy. Such particles both lie at the basis of the universe and form the atoms that make up your body. Ayurveda describes this reality in amazingly similar terms, describing as it does a fundamental field that precipitates as the five elements: space and air (which make up *vata*), fire and water (*pitta*), and water and earth (*kapha*). So when we speak of *vata*, *pitta* and *kapha* we are describing profound and subtle dynamics at the very basis of life.

# THE AYURVEDIC PERSPECTIVE

In Ayurvedic philosophy, the source, or essence, or most fundamental aspect of life, is your "self" – an inner self that operates through your five senses to create the five subtle elements that make up *vata*, *pitta* and *kapha*.

You constantly nourish your mind-body through your interaction with the universe, borrowing atoms to structure your tissues. Your mind-body is organized by a vast intelligence that has its origin in your inner self, and which uses atoms to precipitate into physical matter. On the level of mind you may experience this as, for example, anxiety or joy, which simultaneously in the body precipitate as adrenalin or serotonin.

The intelligence within knows how to generate health. Your body will heal because that is the way it is structured, always trying to return to its template for good health. You have to work hard and put much time and energy into creating the disruptions that bring health problems. But your natural state is to be healthy, which is why it is easier to be healthy than to be ill.

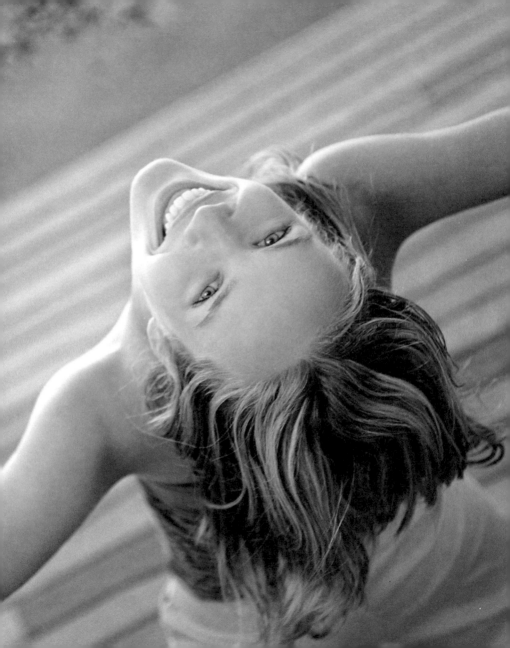

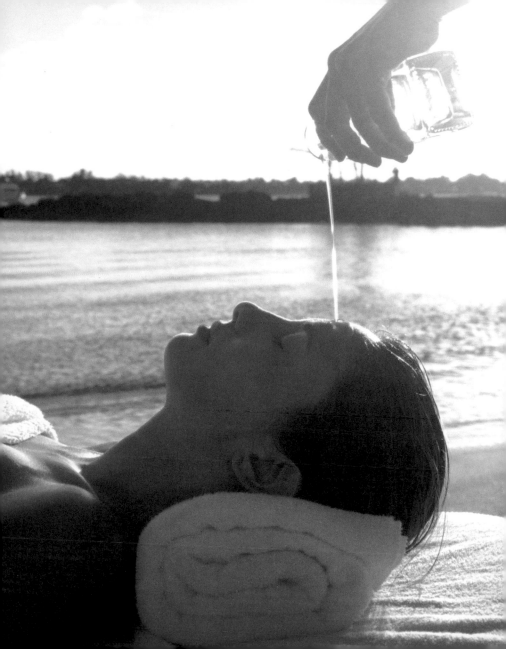

# AYURVEDIC THERAPIES

Ayurveda addresses each person individually: the important point is to make the right choice for you, your circumstances and your imbalances.

An Ayurvedic practitioner, or *vaidya*, will advise changes to your routine, exercise, environment, stressors and so on. In Ayurveda, food is medicine: the *vaidya* will give you information on foods to favour and avoid. She/he may prescribe natural substances such as plant or animal products, minerals and purified metals, in the form of infusions, decoctions, medicated wines, extracts, powders, pills, poultices and oils.

Therapies also include such sophisticated processes as fasting or treatments (*panchakarma*) to eliminate toxins, and a range of tonics to strengthen you. Much of what is prescribed you will do for yourself – a change of routine or exercise. Some things, such as herbal preparations, you will imbibe. You may be advised to take up Transcendental Meditation or yoga, which work in harmony with and are considered part of Ayurveda.

# CREATING HEALTH

Modern medicines work fast. Yet they do not always treat the underlying cause of pain or infection. The healing at a deeper level takes time.

Ayurveda explains why. Food is digested into seven "tissue elements" called *dhatus*. Each of these *dhatus* nourishes particular body tissues. For example, the first *dhatus* produced replenishes our energies, while the second nourishes blood tissues, and so on. These are produced in sequence, one from another, and it takes six to seven days to create each *dhatus*. So a portion of the food you ate almost four weeks ago is still undergoing transformation now to produce a *dhatus* that nourishes your bones, and at the same time some of the food eaten six weeks ago is transforming now to create the *dhatus* that nourishes your reproductive tissues.

If life is disrupted, the quality of nourishment from your digestion is poor and tissues suffer in the same sequence. The body protects deeper tissues by slowing disruptive processes. First energy levels will be lowered, then blood suffers, then muscle, and so on. It depends which tissue is weakest as to where eventual breakdown occurs. It may take up to two years for blood tissues to be significantly disrupted and, say, for anaemia to develop. A few years later, the disease process may impact on muscle and still later on fat tissues. Alzheimer's disease, osteoporosis and infertility may take decades to evolve.

The good news is that this system is much quicker to heal. The body will use the best nourishment generated at each level to create and replenish deeper tissues that are more significant to life and health. If you start to live a better lifestyle and eat healthier foods you begin to create better nourishment immediately. The body will use this better nourishment at each level.

It takes about six weeks for real healing to commence and to be noticed. From then on healing will progress. In our quick-fix culture people often want instant cures, but nature takes time. If you have significant imbalance and health problems you will need to be patient. However, using Ayurveda for better well-being when you are in good health can bring immediate benefits.

# AYURVEDIC DEFINITION OF HEALTH

With *vata*, *pitta* and *kapha* balanced, mind and body work as they were designed to. Food is fully digested, properly absorbed, and readily integrated into tissues. Your body builds perfect new muscles, bones and flesh, and efficiently removes worn-out structures and all toxins. Your body is at its best, energized, strong and stable.

The Ayurvedic concept of health includes the five senses being fully awake, sensitive and refined. The organs of action such as the tongue, hands and feet, eliminatory organs and sex organs work to perfection to fulfill all desires. The senses and the organs of action are coordinated by the mind. A healthy mind means that thoughts are productive and useful, and feelings are true to your nature and are expressions of love and happiness.

So balance of *vata*, *pitta* and *kapha* means excellent digestion and metabolism, fully vital organs of sense and action, and a vibrant, lively mind. And Ayurveda also adds a spiritual dimension to these elements of good health, as discussed in Chapter Three

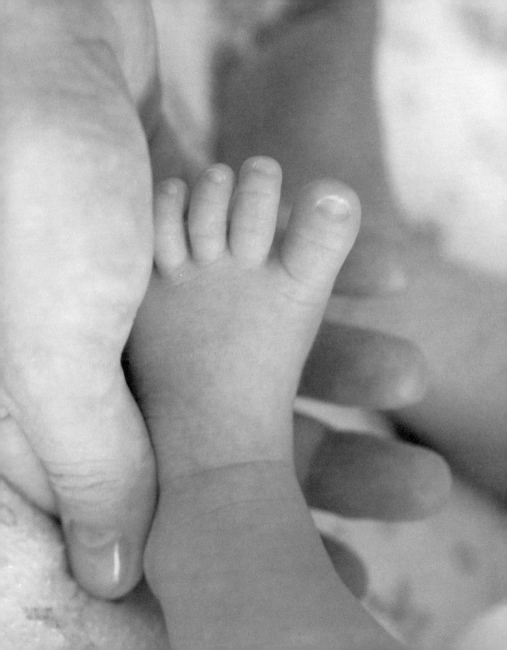

# THE TRUTH OF AYURVEDA

Ayurveda is a very ancient tradition of health, yet its basic principles are resonant of certain fundamental insights that are only now being developed in cutting-edge science. Modern scientific research is beginning the process of validating Ayurveda, and throughout the world in almost all cultures people are now turning to this ancient knowledge. Because it teaches us a way of staying healthy and does not divorce our body from our mind and spirit, nor ourselves from our surroundings, Ayurveda has a profound and widespread appeal to people who are tired of feeling stressed and alienated by many aspects of modern culture.

You will find the principles of Ayurveda to be simple (even deceptively so) and intuitively right. With experience, their true value and usefulness will be appreciated to the full. Ayurveda offers you practical and effective ways to generate health and happiness. The rest of this book is about these insights and how you can apply them in your own life for your benefit and well-being.

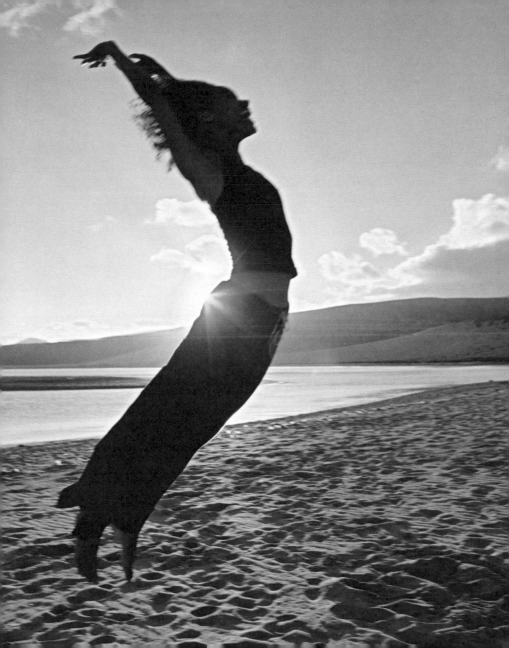

Chapter Two

# the three doshas

The purpose of Ayurveda is health. And just as if we want to keep a plant healthy we nourish the root, so with Ayurveda we nourish the root of life to keep ourselves healthy and happy.

This may seem a difficult concept. There are so many different things that make up our lives, all of which — even the cells in our body — are changing all the time. Ayurveda helps us to understand life by identifying three main "roots" of all activity, three main principles in nature itself.

These three principles, or *doshas*, Ayurveda calls *vata*, *pitta* and *kapha*. Each one of us has a unique natural balance of these three principles, and if that balance is maintained in our everyday lives, we are healthy and happy. If the balance is disturbed, then a lack of ease – disease – may develop.

Ayurveda shows us how to identify our own natural balance of these three *doshas*, and then how to discover the way to keep them in balance.

Probably the most enjoyable way to learn about *vata*, *pitta* and *kapha* is by looking at people. What is a *vata* type of person like, or a *pitta*, or a *kapha*? Which are you, and which are your friends? In this chapter we will take a look at how the three *doshas* make us tick – and we will go on to see how we can use that understanding to create better health.

# WHAT IS VATA?

The first fundamental principle of Ayurveda is *vata*, the dynamic of movement. Everything in your mind and body is on the move, and in Ayurvedic terms, all these movements are due to *vata*. *Vata* causes your limbs to move, powers your circulation, stimulates food to move in your gut – even triggers the thoughts to move in your head. The primary location of *vata* in the body is the pelvis and legs.

*Vata* is like the wind that moves the leaves on the trees and the clouds – yet you do not see the wind. Like the wind, *vata* is described as light, moving and quick; it is irregular, cold, dry and rough. A landscape that is rough and dry and cold will increase your *vata*, as will, similarly, dry weather. *Vata* predominates in the swallow on the wing and the squirrel scurrying in the trees.

*Vata* inspires your enthusiasm and motivates your senses. The flicker of an eyelid and the movement of your tongue in speech are further examples of your *vata* in action. *Vata* gives you speed and vibrancy.

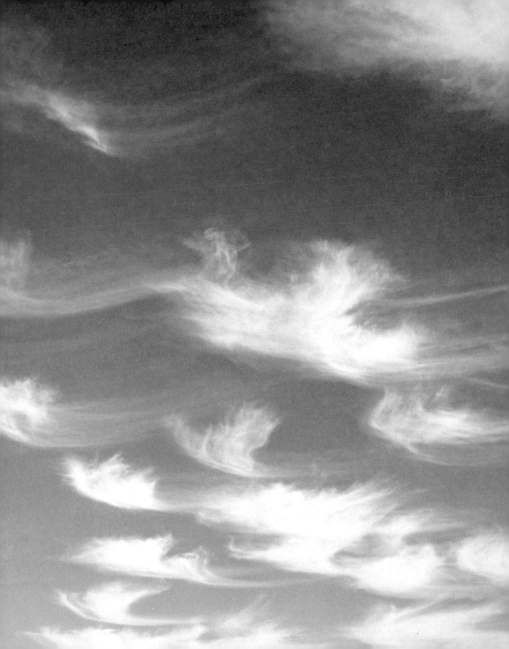

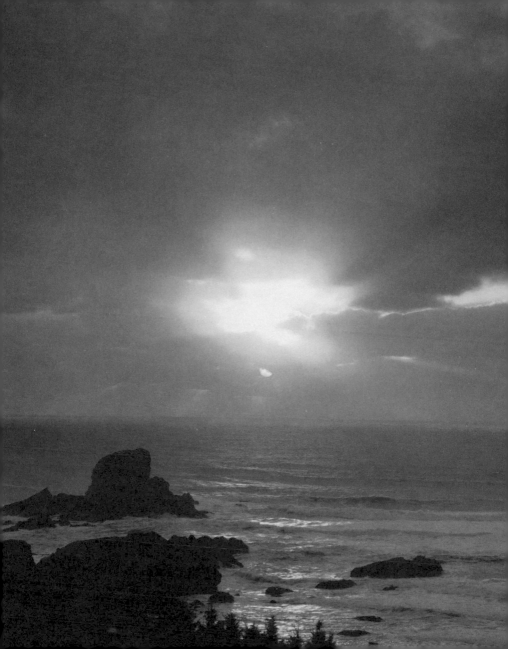

## WHAT IS PITTA?

*Pitta* is the dynamic of transformation. Everything in your mind and body is always being transformed, just as everything is always moving. Transformation is said to be due to *pitta*. Your mind is constantly changing from one thought or feeling to another, and every cell, tissue and organ in the body is undergoing change. Energy is created, old structures deteriorate and are replaced by new ones. The enzymes, hormones and biochemical systems in your body are *pitta* at work. The primary location of *pitta* in the body is the stomach area.

*Pitta* is the fire that transforms things – and like fire, *pitta* is described as having the qualities of being hot, sharp, fluid and light. A hot climate will increase your *pitta*. A hungry lion is dominated by *pitta*.

Fire is associated with light and it is *pitta* that gives the glow of a good complexion. *Pitta* brings warmth to your nature, and in the body is associated with the colours red, yellow and green. *Pitta* is the light that illuminates and transforms life.

# WHAT IS KAPHA?

Where *vata* is responsible for all movements in mind and body and *pitta* is responsible for all transformations, *kapha* is like the glue that holds it all together. *Kapha* is responsible for structure and growth. All the atoms in your body are said to be held together by *kapha*, which integrates all the activities of your mind and body. The primary location of *kapha* in the body is the head, chest and upper portion of the stomach.

*Kapha* has the qualities of being slow, heavy, stable, sticky, soft, cold, oily and sweet. A boggy, dull landscape or weather that is damp and cold will increase your *kapha*. An elephant is an animal with a lot of *kapha*.

*Kapha* is associated with the senses of taste and smell. It nourishes and lubricates, contributing to digestion by providing lubrication in the mouth and stomach. In the nervous system it gives a nourishment sometimes equated with cerebro-spinal fluid. It brings strength, fertility and libido, stamina and resilience. *Kapha* binds all of life together and at its subtlest is love.

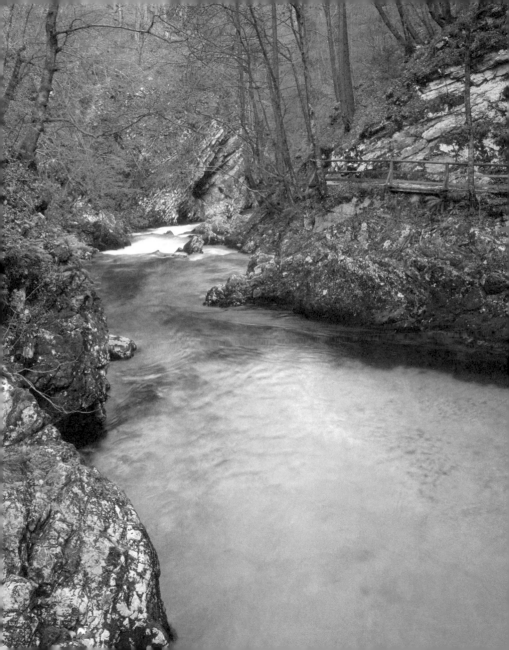

Burrow awhile and build, broad on the roots of things.

ROBERT BROWNING

(1812–1889)

We must learn not to disassociate the airy flower from
the earthy root, for the flower that is cut off from its
root fades, and its seeds are barren, whereas the root,
secure in mother earth, can produce flower after flower
and bring their fruit to maturity.

KABBALAH

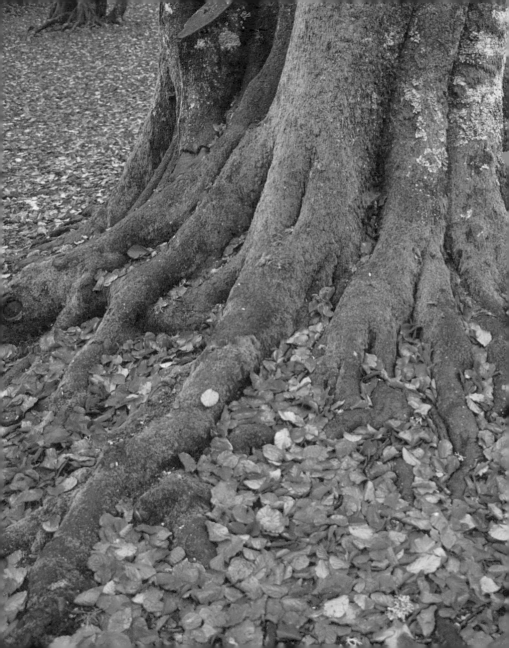

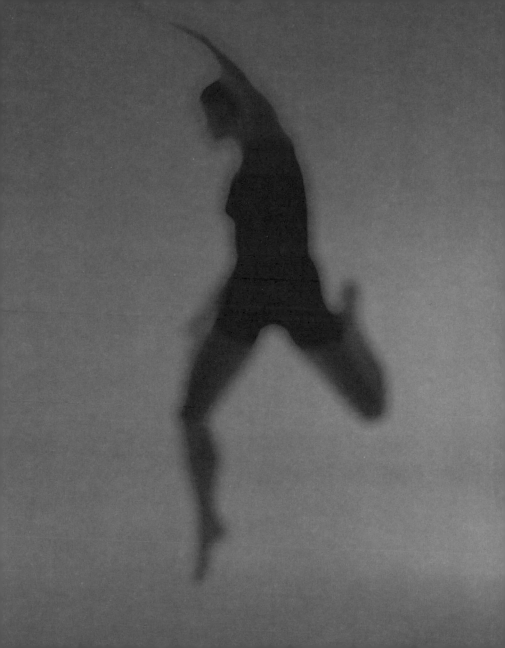

# THE VATA PERSON

*Vata* is about movement, so *vata* people are light, lively and on the move. If you are *vata*, then your body frame is likely to be thin and either tall or short. Gaining weight is not a problem for you. You are refined in feelings, and sensitive – the princess who could not sleep because of the pea in her bed was *vata* in nature. The senses of touch and hearing predominate, so you will love the touch of silk and adore music. Your intuition is good, and you follow your hunches. You are creative and artistic.

Moving fast, *vata* people excel at sprinting and rush from chore to chore. But with a light body frame you do not have stamina, and so tire easily; missing sleep at night does not suit you. Your mind moves fast, thinking quickly and also learning quickly.

If you are *vata*, then you do not like cold – you tend to wrap up well before going out. Your skin and hair may tend to dryness or roughness. *Vata* people can be prone to anxiety, and may talk all day about a near miss in the car, or fret about items lost.

# THE PITTA PERSON

If you have moderate build, strength and stamina, then the chances are you're a *pitta* person. *Pitta* moves at a moderate pace and learns at moderate speed.

*Pittas* are hot-natured, and look warm, with red complexions and perhaps red hair. If you are *pitta*, then a cool evening breeze is refreshing, but the midday sun is too hot. You are passionate about your loved ones, your recreations and your work. You have a sharp appetite: the fire in your stomach demands instant satisfaction.

Your mind is as sharp as your appetite. As the sense of sight predominates, *pitta* people have a good vision, and see a situation clearly. With a strong intellect, you like to understand things and form strong opinions. Order pleases you, and you are a good organizer. Perfectionism is one of your characteristics, and you are competitive and want to win. *Pitta* people are natural leaders.

Delayed in a queue, *pitta* loses patience. A near miss in the car will make you cross with the other driver; if you lose something you won't believe it is your fault.

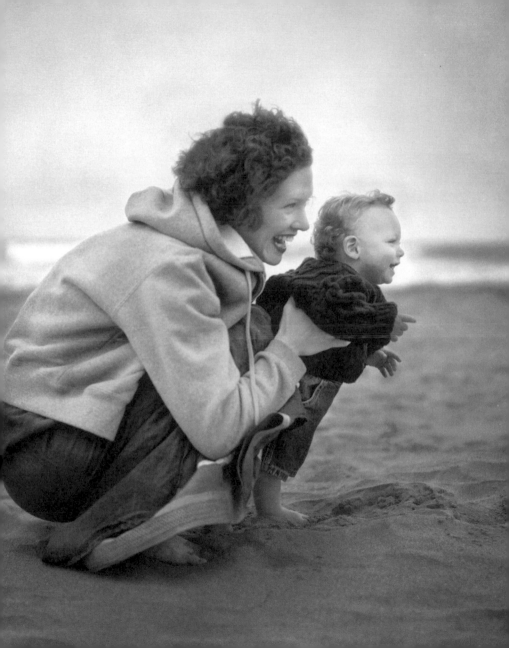

## THE KAPHA PERSON

*Kapha* people are compassionate, kind, stable, strong, ponderous and slow. They have no hope in a sprint, but in a marathon they thrive owing to great stamina. If you are *kapha*, then you probably have a slow metabolism, and so easily put on weight, which you find very difficult to lose. Slowness of mind also causes slowness in picking up information and making decisions. However, you have a long memory, and are never in a rush – your attitude to life tends to be "let's do it tomorrow".

If you are *kapha*, you are grounded and practical. Though slow to change, once change is made you will stick with it. This, along with your strength and stamina, makes you a great achiever. Your stable nature makes you reliable, and a friend for life.

You tend to be of big build, soft-fleshed and with oily skin and hair. The soft nature of *kapha* is compassionate and nurturing.

*Kapha* waits patiently in a queue and is unperturbed by either forgotten items or a near miss in a car.

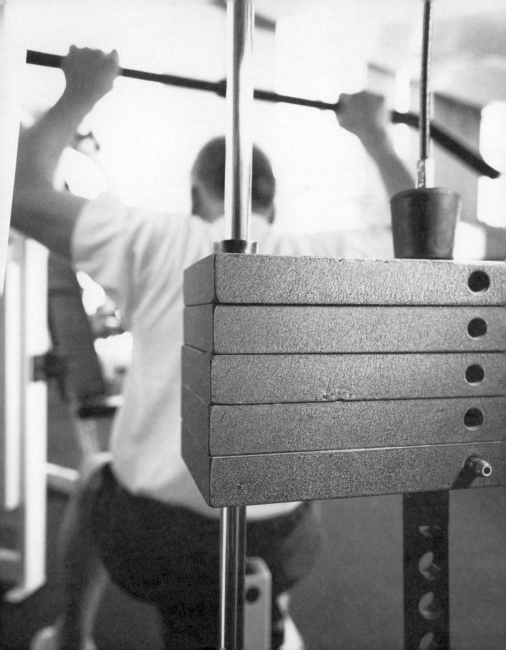

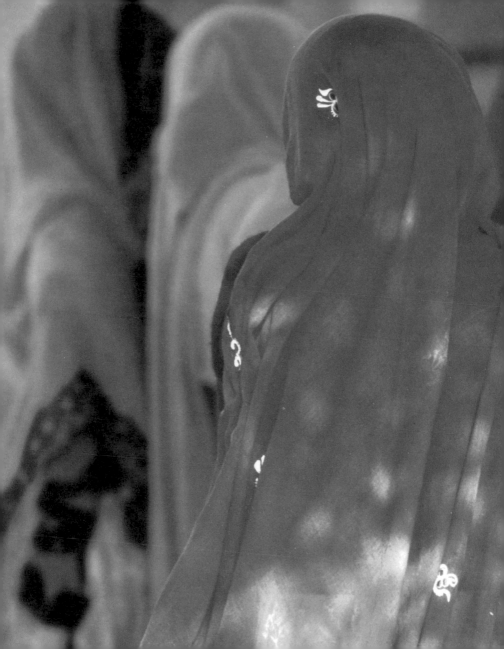

The variety of all things finds a pleasure.

EURIPIDES

(480-406BCE)


Not on one strand are all life's jewels strung.

WILLIAM MORRIS

(1834-1896)

# BALANCE AND IMBALANCE OF VATA

When *vata* is balanced, you have immense inspiration, enthusiasm and vitality. Your creativity thrives, you learn rapidly and your memory is good. Mind and body are integrated; all movements flow with grace and ease.

When out of balance, *vata* can create great problems. Your thoughts – the movements of your mind – may become disturbed by fear, anxiety, panic and insomnia. Inspiration evaporates, and forgetfulness sets in. Bodily aches and pains arise; perhaps constipation occurs.

*Vata* goes out of balance when you choose too many *vata* qualities in life – being in a hurry, living an irregular routine, becoming cold. Thus, as you are drawn to heat when cold, so you should be drawn to opposite qualities to restore your balance. To balance *vata*, get plenty of rest, eat nourishing foods, slow down, live a regular routine, keep warm, have an oil massage. These soothe the moving, light, quick, irregular, rough and dry qualities of *vata*. Anxiety, forgetfulness and other symptoms fade, and feelings of well-being and joy return.

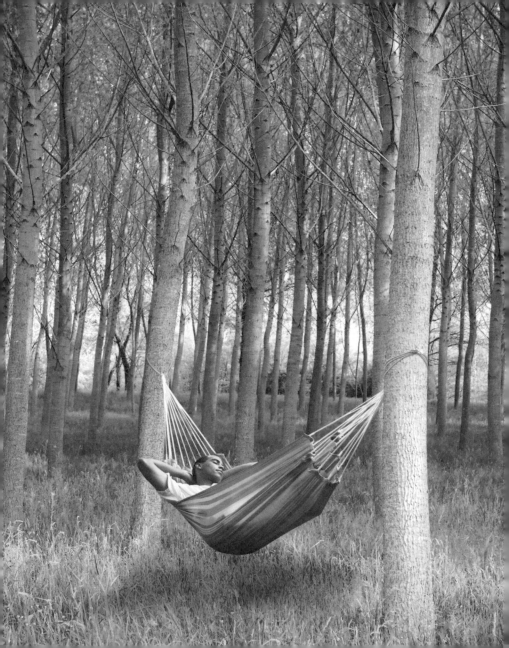

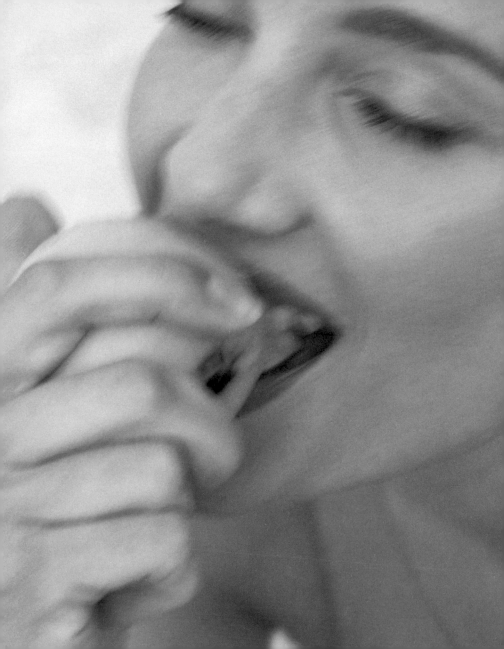

## BALANCE AND IMBALANCE OF PITTA

If you are *pitta*, when balanced you are warm-natured, charming, generous, cheerful and content. You have great physical energy, excellent eyesight and very good digestion. You have a vision for your life, and are enterprising, quick to put things right, neat and precise.

Imbalance of *pitta* causes anger, resentment, jealousy, aggression or obsession, and can lead to physical aspects of overheating such as heartburn, cystitis, diarrhoea, skin rashes, fevers, excess hunger and thirst.

The cause of balance or imbalance lies in everyday choices. If a *pitta* person chooses opposite qualities to his hot, sharp nature, he becomes balanced; if he chooses to overheat by working under pressure, rushing meals, eating curries, drinking a lot of alcohol, over-exercising and getting involved in conflict, he loses balance.

One strategy for balancing *pitta* is to choose foods of a cooling nature – a summer-type diet with salads and fresh fruit. Another is to play. Schedule time for recreation before filling your diary full of work. Chill out!

## BALANCE AND IMBALANCE OF KAPHA

With all the *doshas*, the best of human nature is expressed when they are in balance. *Kapha* people when balanced are strong and stable, with big builds, excellent stamina and a high pain threshold. They are good-natured, even-tempered, generous, kind and compassionate. They are slow to anger and unflappable.

An imbalance of *kapha* means that weight becomes a problem, with cellulite and flab appearing. Heaviness, sluggishness and dullness predominate. Laziness and lethargy set in. Possessiveness and greed manifest themselves. Depression develops. Physical complaints such as coughs, colds, allergies, asthma, diabetes, hypo-thyroidism , greasy skin and sinusitis may also occur.

Sleeping in, eating heavy foods and overeating, being lethargic and slothful, and avoiding exercise and excitement are all choices that unbalance *kapha*. For balance of *kapha* you need to choose the opposite qualities in life. Eat lightly, exercise more, enjoy variety and spice in life, take on challenges, and in general get moving.

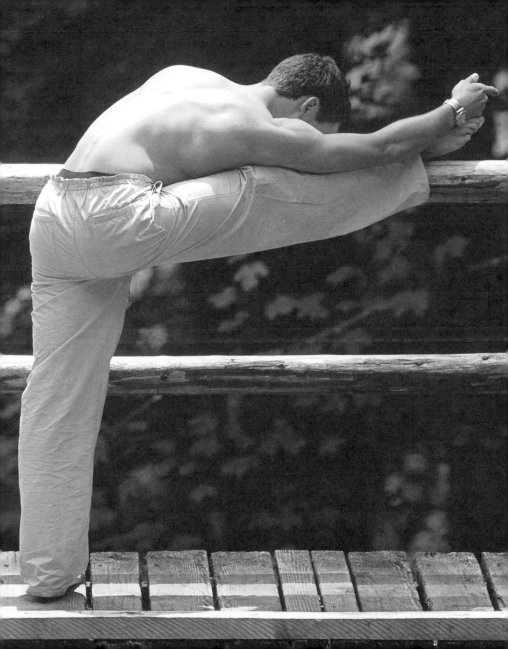

# UNDERSTANDING YOUR NATURE

As you read the descriptions of *vata*, *pitta* and *kapha* you may have felt yourself to be a mixture. This is very likely. Each one of us has our own unique and individual balance of *vata*, *pitta* and *kapha*.

Ayurveda describes seven categories of people according to the predominance of *vata*, *pitta* and *kapha* in their nature. First is a *vata* category where *vata* alone predominates and *pitta* and *kapha* are much less. Similarly there are *pitta* and *kapha* categories. Then there is a *vata-pitta* category where *vata* and *pitta* together predominate and *kapha* is less. An example would be someone of light build who is fast-moving (*vata* qualities), and also very determined and organized (*pitta* qualities). Similarly there are *vata-kapha* and *pitta-kapha* categories. Finally there is the *vata-pitta-kapha* type, with all three equal. People in this last category tend to enjoy excellent health as by nature they are balanced.

To be balanced means to have the right proportion of *vata*, *pitta* and *kapha* for your constitution, or nature, which is determined at conception. If innately you are a *vata-pitta* person with 50 percent *vata*, 40 percent *pitta* and 10 percent *kapha*, then you are balanced when you remain at these proportions. If *vata* increases to 60 percent, it has gone out of balance. So balance does not mean equal proportions of all three *doshas* for everyone.

When you have the correct innate proportion of the *doshas*, you are at your best, in good health and enjoying life. Deviation from the proportion that suits you causes you to suffer. As we have seen, it is the choices you make in life, the way you choose to live life, that result in health or disease, in balance or imbalance.

Ayurveda helps with these choices by allowing you to recognize how you are going out of balance (is it *vata*, *pitta* or *kapha*?). Next it enables you to understand how to regain your health by selecting the opposite qualities in life to the *dosha* that is out of balance. And once you are back to balanced health, Ayurveda will help you to recognize and choose what best suits your nature, enabling you to remain balanced and to express your full potential while enjoying excellent health.

Human subtlety ... will never devise an invention more
beautiful, more simple or more direct than does
Nature, because in her inventions nothing is lacking,
and nothing is superfluous.

LEONARDO DA VINCI

(1452-1519)

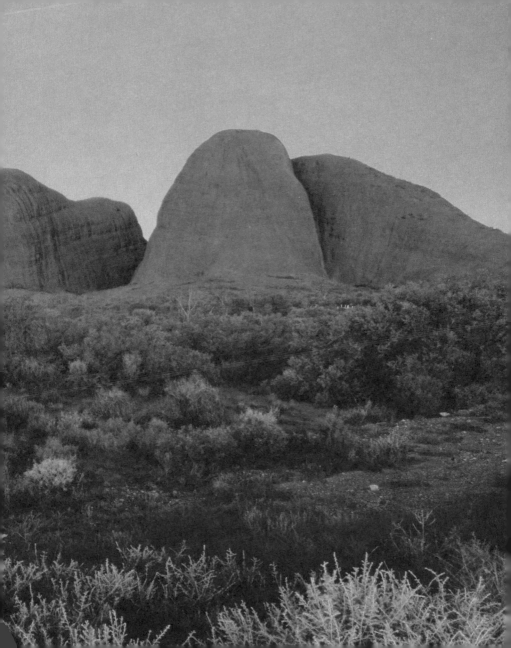

Chapter Three

# the way to health

Ayurveda places great emphasis on digestion and metabolism. These are known as *agnis*, or digestive fires. There are many *agnis*, the main one being in the stomach and small intestine. Ayurveda also discusses seven tissue metabolisms that work in every cell. These get strength from the gut, or gastric, fire. If this is strong, all the tissue metabolisms are active to build strong tissues and keep them healthy.

Every year we replace 98 percent of our atoms, the building blocks of the body; that means that all body tissues are turned over within a few years. Your body is not static: it is an immense flux of constant transformations. If the processes of transformation, the *agnis*, are healthy, then the tissues formed will be strong.

If you are not feeling healthy and energized, you can help yourself simply by beginning to take more care of your digestion so as to balance your *agni*. This will stimulate metabolisms to give more energy and start strengthening your tissues, and after a few months the benefits of improving health will kick in.

Ayurveda recognizes the importance of exercise for health, vitality, strength and stamina. Appropriate exercise improves digestion and metabolism and helps the body cleanse itself of toxins. The Ayurvedic way to health also encompasses strategies to keep you healthy in mind and spirit as well as in your body.

## CARING FOR YOUR DIGESTION

Fundamental to good health is good digestion. For this, you have to cooperate with your digestive system. We abuse ourselves with junk food, eating on the run, eating too much and eating when not hungry, all of which disturb proper metabolism, so that our health suffers.

The single most important thing is to listen to your digestive system. It sends you only one signal about when to eat, and that is – hunger. Eating to be sociable, for comfort or out of boredom disrupts digestion, but such habits are so common that many people rarely experience actual hunger nowadays.

Most weight problems result from being out of touch with your inner needs and nature. If you listen to your gut feeling for food, you will reconnect with that inner intelligence that creates health. By cooperating with it you will gradually normalize your weight, and you will also enjoy your food much more.

Start the day by eating a small breakfast according to your hunger. Not overeating at breakfast will mean that you will then be hungry for a good lunch. Satisfying hunger at lunch without overeating will allow the appetite to return for your evening meal. In between meals have drinks and do not eat unless actually physically hungry. If hungry between meals eat very lightly so as not to rob the hunger from the next mealtime.

This is simple, but it does require a bit of attention. Try developing this new habit: before you eat, first ask "Am I hungry?" Bring your attention to the stomach, where real hunger is felt. And when you finish eating, check your stomach. If you have eaten appropriately you will feel great. If not, there will be a feeling of discomfort or bloating. By simply attending to these signals, you gradually learn how to cooperate. Eating (not overeating) with hunger to satisfy hunger leaves you feeling at your best. Eating the right amount of food at the right time results in health and brings weight to normal.

The best food in the world is no good if you do not digest it properly. Therefore most emphasis is on good digestion. For good digestion the most important thing is to eat according to hunger.

## ENJOYING EATING

Eating should be fun. It is a time to replenish, and the way you do it is important. To be relaxed and happy, always sit to eat. When active, your sympathetic nervous system drives blood to muscles and brain and away from your gut. This happens even when you're watching television or reading, so it is best not to divert attention from your meal. Relax, attend to the food and enjoy it.

If you sit with hunger savouring your food you feel the immense joy of "yummy!" This is the innate signal of good digestion, and should be present every time you eat. Drink sparingly at the meal. A little ginger beforehand with lemon, salt and honey enhances digestion. Such spices as fennel, cumin, coriander and pepper also help. Crucially, these also supply the six tastes – sweet, sour, salty, hot (pepper), bitter (lemon or leafy greens) and astringent (the dry feeling of an apple or dhal). If you do not get all six tastes, you will suffer cravings as the body recognizes that some basic foods are missing. To have all tastes in a meal brings complete fulfilment.

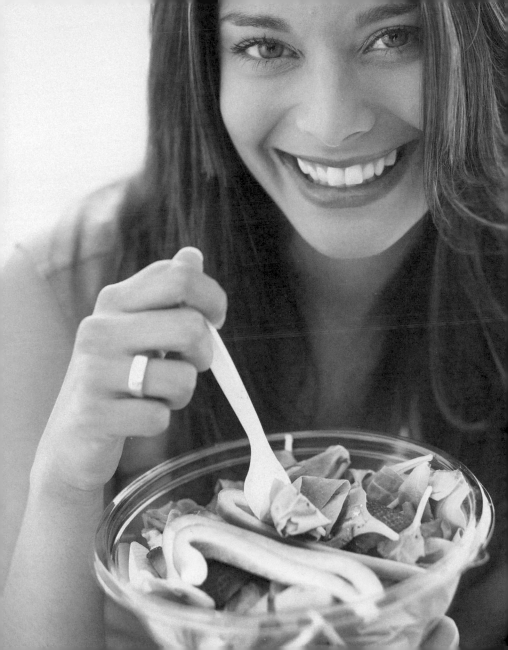

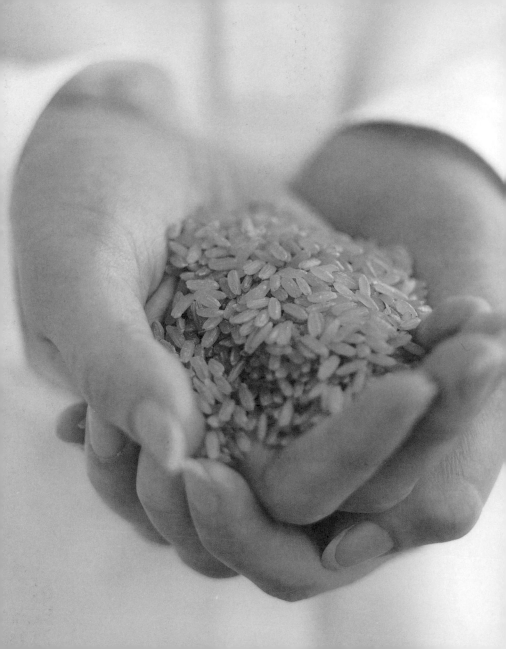

# CHOOSING THE RIGHT FOODS

You are as you eat: choose the best-quality foods according to what needs balancing and according to season. Avoid refined, processed or genetically modified foods.

*Vata* needs hot, nourishing food, and regular meals — three a day plus snacks may be required. Use oils, wheat, rice, quinoa, dairy, nuts and seeds. Spices are good (if not too hot). Beware of leafy greens and pulses, except mung dhal. Choose more of sweet, sour and salty tastes.

*Pitta* digestion is strong: cooler, heavier and blander foods are best. Avoid skipping meals. Suitable foods are sweet fruits, leafy green vegetables, most pulses, unfermented dairy, wheat, barley, oats, rice and sweeteners other than honey. Avoid hot spices such as garlic and chillis. Favour sweet, bitter and astringent tastes.

*Kapha* has a sluggish digestion, so two smaller meals may be enough. Choose steamed, light, hot, dry foods. Grains (except wheat) are good, as is honey (not heated). Use very little oil. Spices are excellent as they stimulate digestion. Hot, bitter and astringent tastes are best.

# EXERCISE FOR VATA TYPES

Exercise must be taken according to your own nature. The light, quick, moving, cold, dry and rough qualities of *vata* increase with exercise. *Vata* types, or people with a *vata* imbalance, should therefore exercise in moderation. *Vata* types tend to get over-enthusiastic: caution is essential as they can get addicted to over-exercising. An example is the over-fit female whose *vata* is so unbalanced that she no longer has a monthly period.

So if you are strong in *vata*, enjoy exercising in moderation. A relaxed walk for 20 to 30 minutes will suit you, or a gentle jog. Try yoga, t'ai chi or Pilates. Since *vata* has little stamina you will do best with exercise that requires bursts of speed with rest periods in between. A 100-metre dash is appropriate. Table-tennis requires speed and agility. *Vata* people are good at gymnastics owing to their refinement and agility. Marathons or extreme sports are definitely not for you.

Having an oil massage before or after more vigorous exercise is an enjoyable way to greater balance.

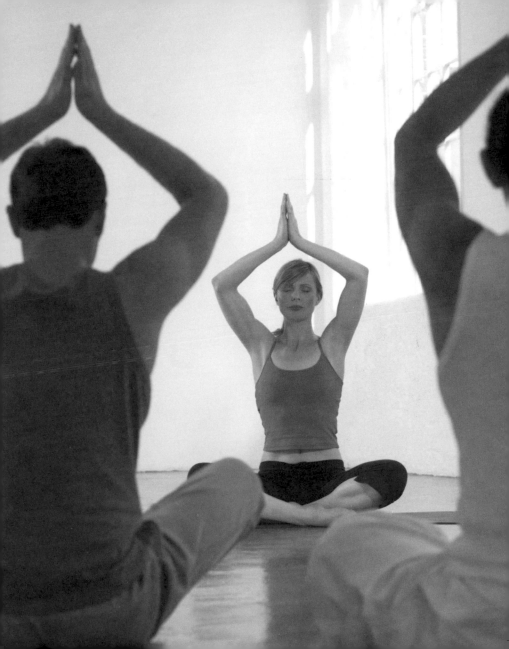

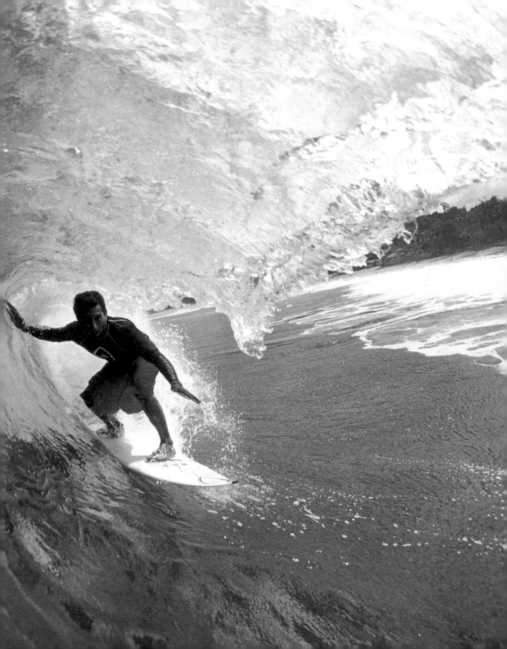

## EXERCISE FOR PITTA TYPES

*Pitta* people have moderate strength and stamina. They also have a very strong competitive spirit and great determination. They make great sportspeople and are often captain of their team.

Sports that suit include tennis, cycling, middle-distance running, car-racing and most team sports. The team element prevents the *pitta* from burning out by trying to do it all himself or herself. In fact, if you are *pitta* and you train vigorously you will easily overheat. For this reason, and because *pitta* is fiery, water sports are appropriate, such as swimming, surfing, windsurfing and sailing. Hill-walking and climbing are good, since its gets cooler as you go higher. Winter sports such as ice-skating and skiing are also suitable.

*Pitta* tends to perspire easily and so has a special need for fluid replacement when exercising. Plain water is best, or alternatively some sweet, *pitta*-reducing fruit juice. Having a coconut-oil massage and a cool shower is a good way to recover from demanding exercise.

# EXERCISE FOR KAPHA TYPES

If you have a predominance of *kapha*, exercise is your best tonic. Exercising near the start of the day can bring amazing benefits to the way you feel and function. Any exercise will be good and in general the more the better.

Since, as a *kapha*, you tend to be stable, strong and slow, exercise for you should be vigorous, demanding, fast and exciting. Marathons are good. Triathlon competitions would also suit. Squash is a fast and vigorous sport. Or join the forward line in a rugby team.

In athletics you have the strength to lift weights and throw the hammer, the discus and the shot. Wrestling is another sport requiring strength (the Sumo wrestler is definitely a *kapha* type). Skydiving and hang-gliding introduce you to the space element, which will balance *kapha*'s predominance of earth and water elements.

Exercise at any time of the day and in any season is good for *kapha*. Without adequate exercise *kapha* people put on too much weight and can easily become dull and despondent. For *kapha* people exercise is a must.

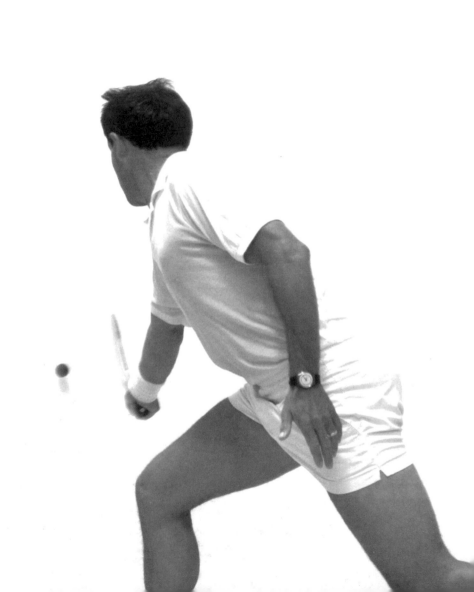

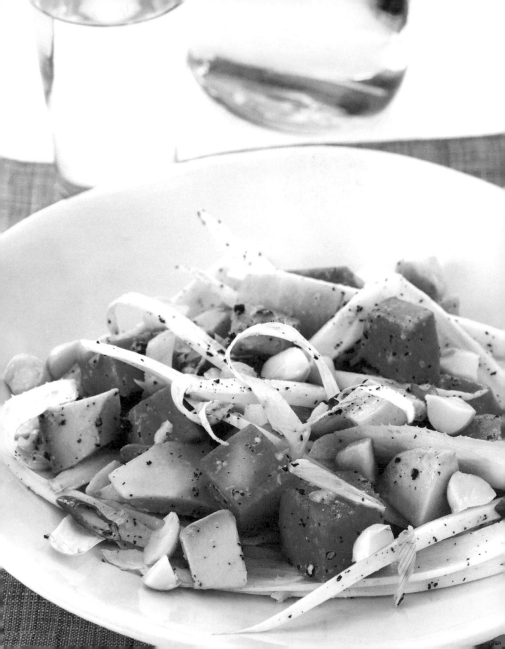

Tell me what you eat: I will tell you who you are.

JEAN-ANTHELME BRILLAT-SAVARIN

(1755–1826)

When diet is wrong, medicine is of no use.
When diet is right, medicine is of no need.

AYURVEDIC PROVERB

# THE STAGES OF DISEASE

Illness stems from an imbalance of the *doshas*, and Ayurveda describes six stages in the development of disease. An excess of a *dosha* builds up in its own location; secondly it gets agitated; thirdly it spreads through the body; fourthly it settles in a vulnerable area. At the fifth stage disease manifests, while at the sixth stage complications of the disease occur. There are symptoms from the first stage – mild at the start, but enough to make you aware that all is not right. At stages two and three you are worried; by stage three or four you may visit your doctor.

It is important to take action at the early stages of disease development, yet these are the stages that conventional medicine will not diagnose. From stages one to three the process is easier to reverse, while at stage four the seeds of disease are germinating but still easy to root out. Stage five is late in the day: the condition will need stronger treatment to reverse, which is why medicines often have such side-effects. With Ayurveda you can prevent disease and effect healing at earlier stages.

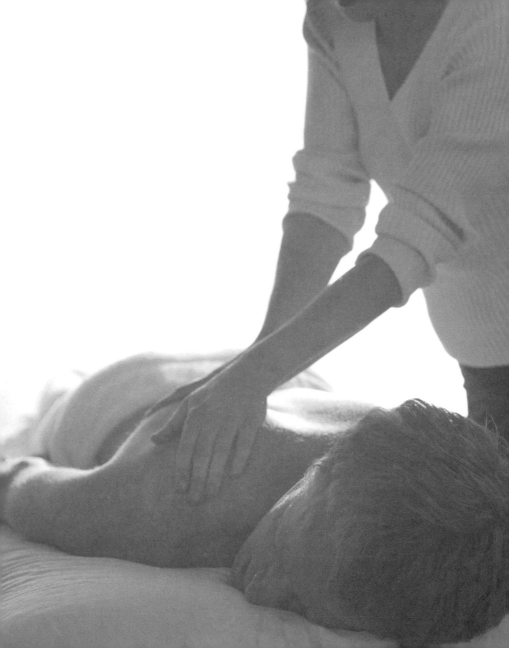

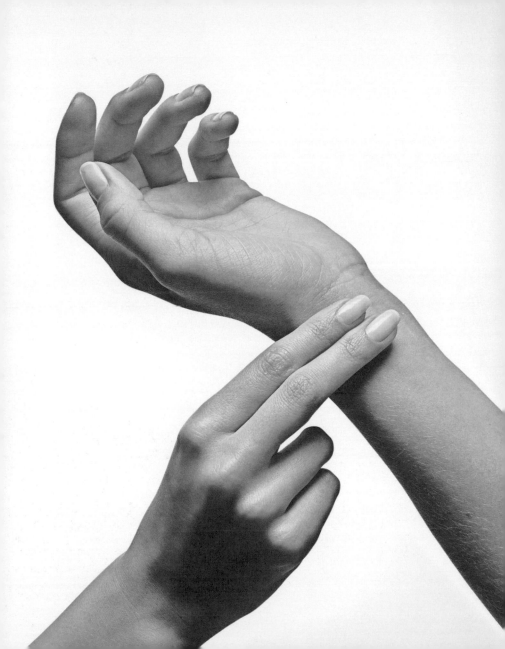

## SEEING A PRACTITIONER

From the moment you arrive at the clinic of an Ayurvedic practitioner, or *vaidya*, she/he observes you closely. Your structure and stance, how you move, think and talk, your sense of humour – all speak of your *vata*, *pitta* and *kapha*. She/he will question you on current and past health problems, and on all aspects of your lifestyle.

The *vaidya* is likely to examine your tongue and will always take your pulse. The pulse is an important part of Ayurvedic diagnosis as it reflects the qualities of *vata*, *pitta* and *kapha* and their balance in the body.

The practitioner thus establishes your state of health, your imbalances and their causes. She/he may advise you to make changes – in lifestyle, food, exercise, attitude or feelings – offer you ways to cope with stress and to enliven digestion, and suggest mechanisms to eliminate toxins and herbs to heal or strengthen. At the first consultation you are likely to discuss a plan involving just a few changes: in future consultations you can evolve your programme and improve your health further.

# STRATEGIES OF TREATMENT

In Western medicine, a consultation is almost always wholly disease-oriented: the doctor analyzes the disease and tries to understand what specific part of what tissue or organ is involved. The process is very specialized. By contrast, an Ayurvedic consultation is more generalized and holistic. Instead of looking for a specific localized problem, Ayurveda looks to universal dynamics operating everywhere in your mind-body – the *doshas* – the balancing of which cures all the specific problems.

Therefore, rather than just using medicines to treat disease, Ayurveda uses a fourfold strategy. The first stage is to identify and put a stop to whatever is disturbing the *doshas* – the foods, activities, recreations, and so on, that do not suit you. The next is to introduce opposite qualities to the disturbed *dosha* to reverse the disease process: this might be, for example, cooling foods and activities for an overheated *pitta*. Then Ayurveda will use effective herbal and mineral medicines that balance specific functions and act as tonics to vulnerable parts.

These may have side benefits but never harmful side-effects. Finally, where the strength of the disease warrants it, Ayurveda resorts to strong treatments such as *panchakarma* (elimination of toxins) and the use of processed metals in herbal medicines.

Ayurveda further differs from conventional medicine in that a primary purpose of the practitioner, or *vaidya*, is to help you to heal by enlightening you and enabling you to make better life choices. In medicine, the doctor treats and the patient heals. Ayurveda, by contrast, empowers you to heal yourself. The *vaidya* also uses his or her knowledge to select appropriate *panchakarma* treatments and herbal and mineral supplements and tonics to aid healing.

Although different, Ayurveda is totally integrative with conventional medicine. However, the full ranges of Ayurvedic treatments are not always available and it is advisable to seek a medical diagnosis if you have a disease. When you know what the problem is you can use Ayurveda along with the medicines from your doctor, and choose advice that helps you to heal.

# ELIMINATING TOXINS

Ayurveda gives the name *ama* to all toxins that arise in your mind-body. *Ama* occurs when digestion or any other process of transformation goes wrong. This *ama* is deposited in cells and tissues, disrupting them and causing disease. Your body has mechanisms for keeping itself clean and free of such debris. Disease begins when these mechanisms fail to clear the accumulations.

There are several ways to prevent and eliminate *ama*. First is to stimulate digestion. Ginger, fennel, cumin, coriander, cinnamon, cloves and black pepper aid digestion and prevent *ama* formation. Spices and herbs that help to break down *ama* include ginger, turmeric, basil and fenugreek. One purpose of many Ayurvedic herbal preparations is to clear *ama* from your tissues.

Exercise stimulates your body's functions and clears *ama*. This is why stiffness and sluggishness disappear with a morning walk. Another strategy is a fast: for *vata* a very light fast; for *pitta* a moderate fast; and for *kapha* a significant fast. It is good for all to eat lightly one day a month, taking only soups, fruit and fluids. Sipping hot water through the day flushes out toxins from your body.

The branch of Ayurveda devoted to detoxing is called *panchakarma*. Water-soluble toxins are eliminated via your kidneys, but toxins that dissolve in oils or fats are harder to get rid of and gather in your tissues. Many fat-soluble chemicals now pollute our food and environment, which may contribute to serious illnesses.

*Panchakarma* may provide one solution to this modern problem. Treatments involve taking oils by mouth and massage until body tissues are saturated. Then follow heat treatments – steam baths or hot oil massages. Finally comes the cleansing of a purgative or enema. This process extracts the fat-soluble toxins from your cells and draws them to the gut, from where they are eliminated. Such treatments are burgeoning around the world in health spa facilities. They are strong treatments requiring a great deal of rest and a very light diet.

Some elimination of toxins is needed in the treatment of almost all illness, so this forms another important facet of the Ayurvedic approach to health.

# MASSAGE

Massage nourishes feelings, eases pain, soothes mental tensions, prevents fatigue, lubricates muscles and joints and gives strength. Ayurveda advises a daily massage. A beautiful tradition is to massage babies and children.

On rising, give yourself an oil massage as part of your morning routine. Use sesame oil (sunflower or coconut oil if you are strong in *pitta*). Massage from the head down, with circular movements on joints and straight ones on the limbs. On the stomach, starting from the right hip, do circles coming up on your right side, across under the ribcage and down on your left. Leave the oil on for 10 minutes and then enjoy a hot bath or shower.

*Vata* moves *pitta* and *kapha*, and sesame oil is the best substance to balance *vata*, so that after this massage all three *doshas* will move appropriately in your mind-body. Within 10 minutes of applying sesame oil it can be measured in the bloodstream and so is available to all your tissues, providing excellent nourishment and helping to prevent ageing.

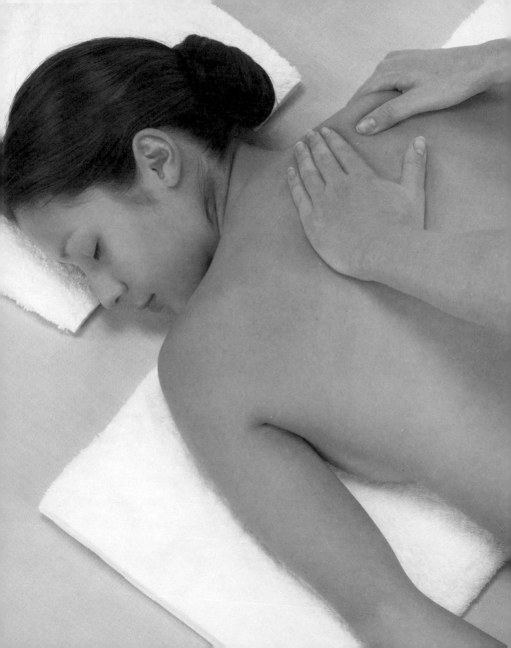

# HERBS AND TONICS

Ayurvedic practitioners respect herbs and know their qualities, tastes, energies, post-digestive effects and specific effects in the body. Ayurveda describes the healing properties of thousands of plants; scientific research exists on the benefits of about 500 of these.

Common Ayurvedic herbs you will now find in health-food stores include Ashwagandha (*Withenia somnifera*), the best anti-stress herb; Brahmi (*Bacopa moniera*), for memory; and Guggulu (*Balsamedendron mukul*), for arthritis, high cholesterol and obesity.

A herb can have many effects on your body. The *vaidya* must choose the specific combination that is best for you. For example, if you suffer from a hot, moist eczema he or she prescribes a cool, drying preparation, thereby establishing a healing relationship between living beings. Ayurveda differs from herbal medicine in that it uses also animal products, minerals and purified metals, and in that it uses complex combinations of ingredients as opposed to single herbs. The *vaidya* will

combine some herbs to support digestion and metabolism, others to eliminate toxins, others to treat *vata*,
*pitta* or *kapha*, others for your problem and yet others to
counteract any possible side-effects. There may be up to
40 ingredients. The recipes for most of the commonly
used preparations were written down thousands of years
ago. There are many different forms – powders, pills,
pastes, decoctions, medicated wines and herbalized oils.

A medicine generally contains one active chemical.
An Ayurvedic preparation may contain hundreds of
active chemicals working together in a complex synergy.
Therefore the concentrations of active principles are
minuscule in comparison to a medicine and they work in
a completely different way. Side-effects are rare.

Two types of herbal are described in Ayurveda. One
treats disease and restores balance. The other enhances
health and vitality and is especially useful in preventing
the adverse effects of ageing. One such, Amrut Kalash,
has been shown to be the best antioxidant ever studied,
enhancing the immune system and protecting against
factors contributing to heart disease and stroke.

Harmony is eating and resting, sleeping and waking:
balance in all you do. This is the path to peace.

BHAGAVAD GITA

(6TH CENTURY BCE)

Still glides the Stream, and shall for ever glide;
The Form remains, the Function never dies.

WILLIAM WORDSWORTH

(1770–1850)

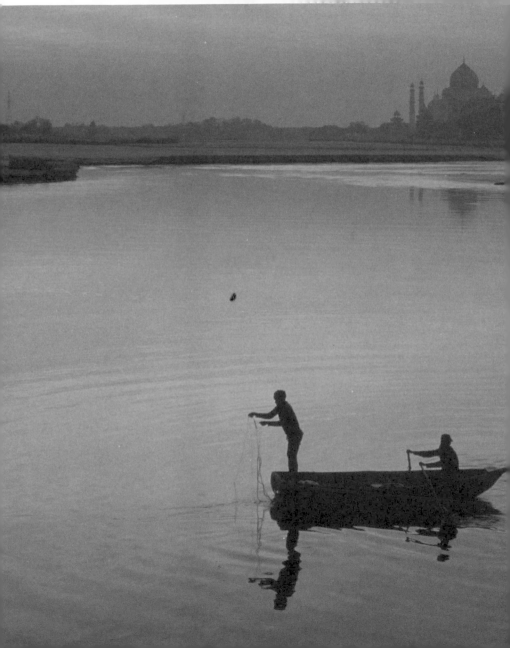

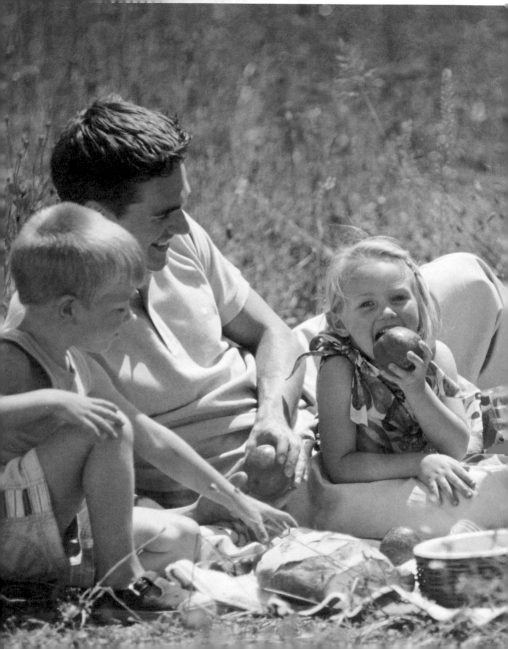

# HEALTH OF MIND

Three fundamental Ayurvedic principles govern the mind: *sattva*, *rajas* and *tamas*. *Sattva* is purity of mind and implies all virtues, such as courage, wisdom, honesty and love; *sattva* is mental health. *Rajas* is excess activity – stress, egoism, aggression, anger, hate. *Tamas* is dullness, lethargy, depression, greed and stagnation.

*Tamas* increases with stale, old, recooked, greasy, processed foods, potatoes, mushrooms and overeating. *Rajas* increases with coffee and other stimulants, garlic, onions, vinegar, chillis, pickles, salt, highly spiced food, alcohol and fizzy drinks. Red meat increases both.

To improve mental health, enhance *sattva*. All the healthy routines, digestive advice, and nourishing experiences described in this book will help. Choose better foods: *sattva* is enhanced by a light diet including seasonal fruits and vegetables; grains and lightly roasted nuts and seeds; dairy products in moderation; and some spices. Foods cooked with love and eaten with settled mind in a settled atmosphere generate *sattva*.

# BODY, MIND AND SPIRIT

When *vata*, *pitta* and *kapha* are balanced, your body is in good health. The Sanskrit word for health is *swastha*, and its meaning introduces a spiritual dimension to the understanding of health. *Swastha* literally translates as "established in the self". The concept of self in Ayurveda goes beyond what we usually conceive our "self" to be. Ayurveda recognizes you – each one of us – to be the total potential that structures the whole universe.

From the Ayurvedic point of view, your mind is like a vast ocean that has waves of great activity on the surface, but profound stillness at its depth. This deep stillness it describes as pure consciousness, silent wakefulness beyond even the faintest thought. Just as a wave draws its strength, vitality and very existence from its source in the ocean, so your mind draws its creativity, intelligence and energy from pure consciousness deep within.

In Ayurveda, a healthy mind means being aware of the connectedness of your own inner consciousness and the universe around you. Your mind is integrated, and you draw the innate potential of your own vast intelligence, energy, creativity, love and joy, and project it into your environment.

But there is more still to the Ayurvedic understanding, a bigger perspective that lets us glimpse a remarkable state of health for ourselves and for the world as a whole. Ayurveda regards the ocean of consciousness that creates your mind and body as also being the creator of all other waves on the ocean – the whole of the physical universe. Everything that exists in the universe is waves from the same source – the galaxies, our solar system, a rainforest, your house, you. Ayurveda gives practical guidelines on how to keep all the elements in balance.

Why is awakening your spiritual source important for your health? By being integrated with your source within, you are in touch with the same source that manifests as the universe around you. Spontaneously your feelings, thoughts, speech and actions are appropriate for your surroundings, harmonious, wise and loving. This is the basis of spiritual living. A life lived in love, wisdom, integration, success and health is implied by *swastha*.

## NURTURING YOURSELF

Life never stands still. You become either more or less healthy from day to day. Ayurveda teaches the joy of constantly creating better health.

Through food, tonics and exercise you nurture yourself. You also digest and metabolize everything you hear, touch, see, taste and smell. Ayurveda cautions that for health in mind and body, you expose your senses only to uplifting, nourishing experiences.

Good speech and behaviour act as tonics. The concept of health concerns wholeness. Your relationship with your whole universe determines your health. Every feeling, thought, speech and action, every incoming sensation, every morsel of food, all should be wholesome.

Take responsibility for your thoughts and feelings. If you persist in negative and unproductive thoughts and feelings you are choosing to disturb your health. Negative patterns can be changed with a bit of effort. Strategies exist in other aspects of Vedic knowledge to help here. But do choose to love as much as possible. Love heals.

In fact, the whole ethos of Ayurveda is love. You must learn to love yourself. This implies attending to, listening to and cooperating with your own nature and needs. Eat when hungry, rest when tired, enjoy positive experiences and love. We often get out of touch with ourselves because we are so focused on our environment.

If someone says that to listen to your own needs is selfish, they are unwise. A tenet of many cultures is to love your neighbour as yourself – which means loving yourself as much as your neighbour. We often make demands of ourselves we would never ask of anyone else.

One further element of self-nurturing is the most fundamental of all and empowers you to achieve spontaneously all other strategies of Ayurveda. Allow all waves of thought to settle, and awaken the stillness of your own ocean of consciousness – your inner self. The best way to achieve this is through Transcendental Meditation, an ancient Vedic tradition that is also the only scientifically verified meditation technique. Regularly done, this settling down of the mind results in a transformation toward ideal health, happiness and fulfilment.

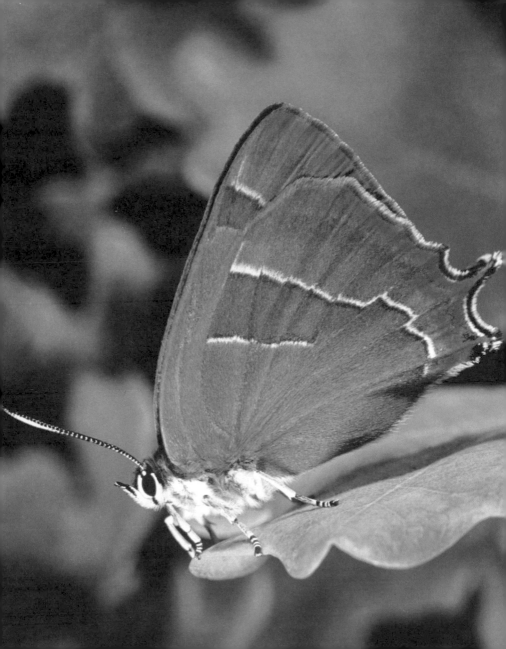

Life belongs to the living, and he who lives must be
prepared for change.

JOHANN WOLFGANG VON GOETHE

(1749-1832)

First say to yourself what you would be; and then do
what you would have to do.

EPICTETUS

(c.55-c135CE)

Chapter Four

# the ayurvedic cycles

There is a cyclical rhythm to life. We observe the cycles of day and night, of the seasons of the year and of our own life. Ayurveda describes these cycles in terms of *vata*, *pitta* and *kapha*. The key to health is to maintain our balance amid the changing phases.

Let us consider the cycle of life. The first 20 years is the *kapha* phase. *Pitta* predominates between 20 and 60. And over the age of 60, *vata* takes over. These different phases have important implications for health. The principles of *vata*, *pitta* and *kapha* give us insight into why we are drawn to certain things at certain times, and how to keep our balance.

The year is also divided into *kapha*, *pitta* and *vata*

phases. The cold, damp, heavy weather of winter along with the spurt of growth in spring are both due to *kapha* predominance. The *pitta* quality of heat predominates in summer. The autumn, with its cooler breezes, is *vata* time of year.

Traditional societies were adjusted to their environment, cultivating balance in life. Today, disconnected from nature around us, we are disconnected from our own nature and imbalance is cultivated. For example, our whole nature changes with the arrival of winter, yet we think that a thick coat and central heating are all we need. Ayurveda helps us recognize how to keep our balance as we change with the seasons.

# KAPHA IN THE CYCLE OF LIFE

It may seem odd that childhood is the *kapha* phase of life, as children are light, quick, moving – all *vata* qualities. But *kapha* is responsible for growing and structuring tissues and so predominates at an early age. Children tend to do naturally the right things to keep balanced. They get up early, keep busy, run about and like excitement, balancing *kapha* though seeming to express *vata*.

If parents or carers do not realize this, they may act in ways detrimental to a child's well-being. If a child is allowed to sleep in, is fed ice cream or yogurt straight from the refrigerator and is not encouraged to exercise, *kapha* goes out of balance, and the child suffers. *Kapha* predominates in the head and chest: many childhood ailments are *kapha* types of problem in a *kapha* part of the body. Tonsillitis, coughs and colds are *kapha* out of balance. Allergies and asthma involve *kapha*.

Children need variety, exercise, warm, nourishing foods, and to rise early. Such *kapha*-balancing strategies will build strong structures for a healthy future.

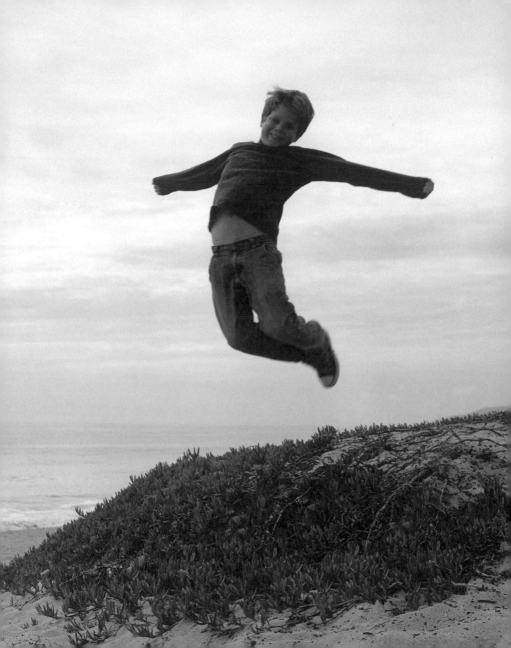

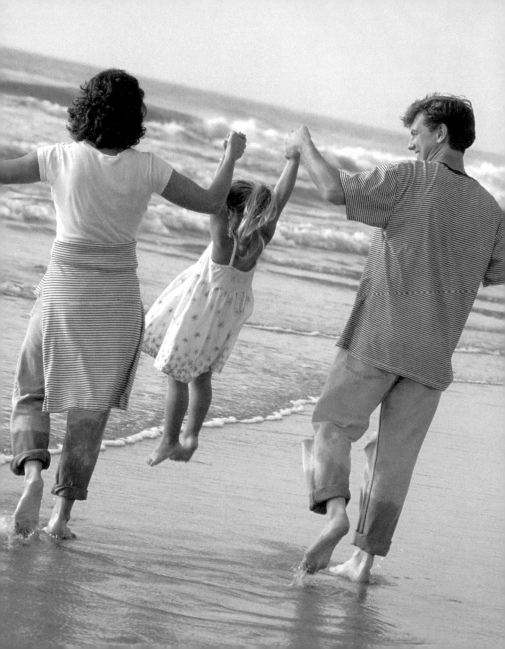

# PITTA IN THE CYCLE OF LIFE

Having built a strong foundation for life, we move into *pitta* phase at the age of 20, which lasts until we are 60. *Pitta* brings ambition, determination and the necessary organizational skills to achieve our aims in life.

Knowing this, you can live so as to prevent problems. Avoid factors that increase and disturb *pitta*, such as rushing, taking on too much, creating friction at work and home, eating rushed meals without true hunger, and imbibing too many hot-natured substances such as alcohol and chillis. If there is strong *pitta* in your nature, you are now even more prone to imbalance.

*Pitta*'s main location is from the chest to the navel; other important locations are the skin and eyes. Now we see growing incidences of such complaints as ulcers, heartburn, colitis, dermatitis and inflammations: *pitta* problems in *pitta* parts of the body. At the end of this phase of life many people have started using glasses.

The most important strategy at this phase of life is to balance work and play. Play with your children!

# VATA IN THE CYCLE OF LIFE

The *vata* time of life begins at 60, and is the time when people are attracted to balancing *vata*. *Vata* is quick, moving, cold, dry, rough and irregular, and so is balanced by the opposite qualities. Ways to do this include maintaining a regular routine, having warm foods and drinks, taking gentle exercise, keeping warm, going to bed early, and perhaps enjoying an afternoon rest. Elders do not generally enjoy excess noise, excitement or strain, and naturally tend to take life easier.

With *vata* imbalance, which happens especially easily for a *vata* type at this time, many problems arise. *Vata* locations are below the navel, the bones, the nervous system and the sense of hearing. Discomforts suffered by older people are mainly *vata* (movement) problems, occurring in *vata* locations. Examples include constipation, incontinence, prostate problems, osteoporosis (lightness and thinness of bones are *vata* qualities), forgetfulness, Alzheimer's disease, Parkinson's disease, strokes and deafness.

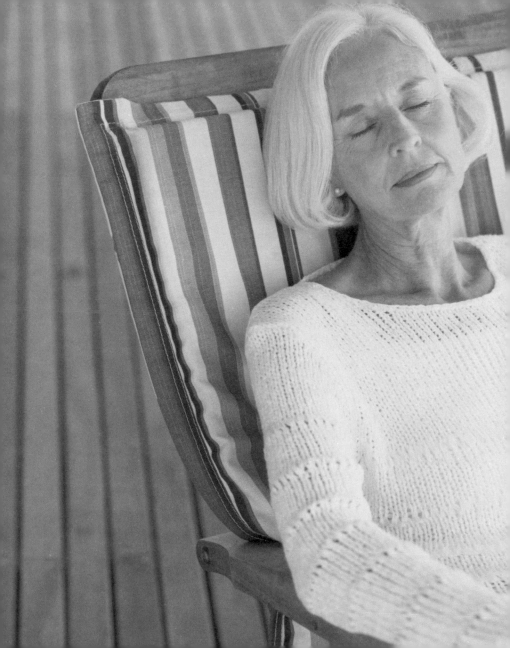

Living creatures are nourished by food, and food is
nourished by rain; rain itself is the water of life, which
comes from selfless worship and service.

BHAGAVAD GITA

(6TH CENTURY BCE)

You cannot step twice into the same river, for other
waters are continually flowing in.

HERACLITUS

(c.540–c480BCE)

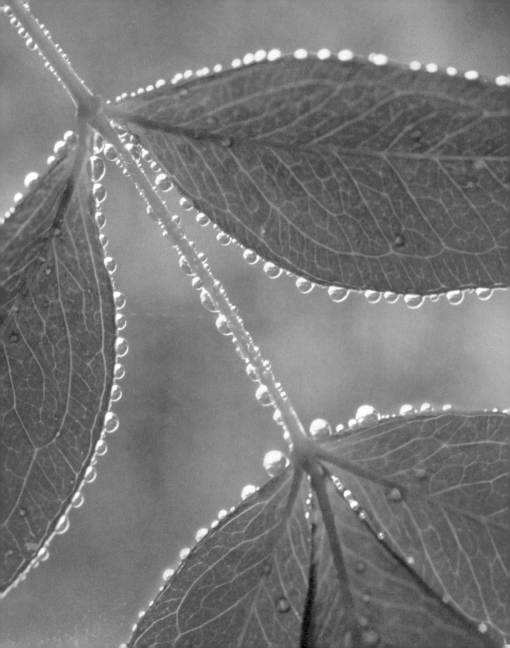

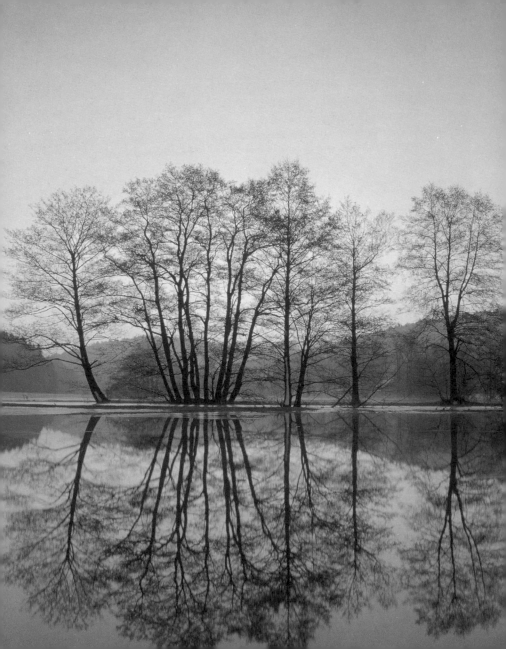

# KAPHA IN THE CYCLE OF THE YEAR

Ayurveda sees both the dull, damp, cold winter and the growth and energy experienced in spring as reflecting a *kapha* time of year, since the winter qualities are those of *kapha*, while growth also is a function of *kapha*.

Traditionally during the winter season people would start working to prepare for the spring. Nowadays really vigorous, energetic training and sports still take place in winter and spring, such as weight training, squash, cross-country running and rugby football. Now we feel the need for warm food and drink to balance the cold of *kapha*. Variety and spice in life is essential during *kapha* time of year to lighten up dull, cool days.

If you do not favour such *kapha*-reducing strategies in winter you will be prone to *kapha* problems, all the more so if there is a great deal of *kapha* in your nature. The results could range from seasonal affective disorder (SAD – the winter blues) or colds and coughs, to a tendency to put on weight. In the spring, a problem may be hayfever. All these involve *kapha* imbalance.

# PITTA IN THE CYCLE OF THE YEAR

Traditional festivals were often held at the end of a season, enabling us to adjust for the coming one. Festival or not, over a two-week period we should alter our routine and foods to those suited to the season about to start.

Although this Ayruvedic advice is rarely followed today, we still recognize that in summer we desire cooler foods and drinks. We naturally wish to take time out to enjoy. We take our holidays. The sea or the lakes are a popular summer destination, and this innate desire to chill out and to be by water is natural for balancing the hot and fiery *pitta*. An understanding of Ayurveda allows us to do this even better. For example, we can choose more wisely the *pitta*-reducing foods.

By using Ayurveda we can avoid problems that may start to emerge toward the end of summer owing to *pitta* going out of balance. *Pitta* people have to be especially careful to keep their balance in summer, otherwise they will suffer anger, irritability or other mental or physical inflammations, even fever, in autumn.

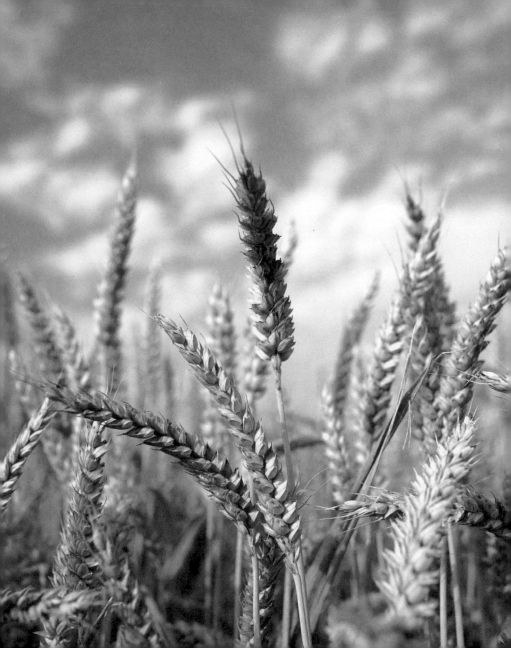

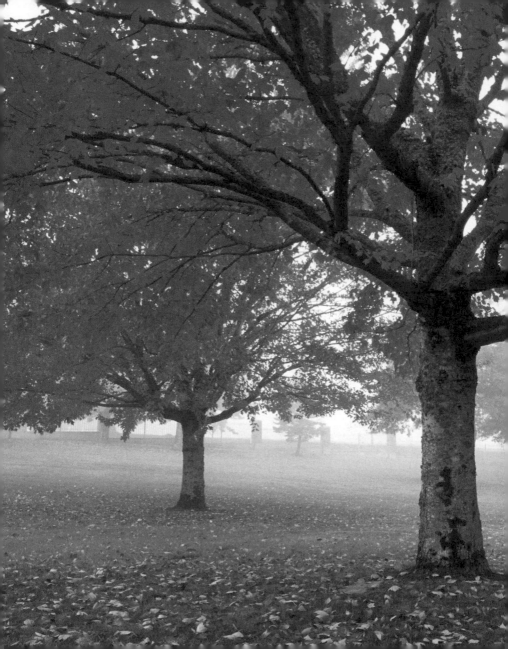

# VATA IN THE CYCLE OF THE YEAR

*Vata* season, autumn, is the time to replenish, as nature does. *Vata* is movement, and rest is ideal for its balance. Now is the time to take life easy – to cut back on activities, go to bed earlier, take weekends off, have massages, soak in hot baths and turn to hot, nourishing foods.

However, this is not what happens. For children and teachers it is back to school. Many people start evening classes or a new activity. Toward Christmas we go manic: partying, shopping, organizing gifts, writing endless cards and generally overdoing it. Imbalance results in misery. But this season is wonderful if you are balanced.

Christmas is a fascinating festival. It comes at the end of the *vata* season to remind us to balance *vata* and change our ways toward balancing *kapha* for the winter to come. Warmth, comfort, family, friends and heavy foods are all influences to settle *vata*. After some days of heavy foods we start wanting to get out for a bit of exercise. Then we party in the new year. In this way we move from balancing *vata* to balancing *kapha* over this time.

# THE CYCLE OF THE DAY

Opposite qualities bring balance. Ayurveda informs us how to know clearly what suits us at what time, with regard not only to the seasons of the year but also to the time of day. In this way Ayurveda empowers us to better keep our balance.

The day is divided into two 12-hour cycles. *Kapha* comes up from 6am to 10am and also between 6pm and 10pm. *Pitta* is there from 10am to 2pm and also from 10pm to 2am. Finally *vata* is up from 2pm until 6pm and again from 2am to 6am. So the day – and also the night – is a *kapha-pitta-vata* cycle.

The cycle of day starts at 6am. This might come as a shock to some, but before our grandparents' generation, it was usual to get up and go to bed with the sun. Our bodies have an innate "circadian" rhythm, which operates roughly on a 24-hour cycle and reacts to light and dark. Many of us nowadays ignore this "body clock", because electricity allows us to stay up late – and with that, conversely, comes the tendency to sleep in.

Sleep is heavy, slow, stable, solid and soft. So is *kapha*. Therefore to sleep in is to add *kapha* qualities to *kapha* time of the day. The result is that you feel heavy and dull after sleeping in, because your *kapha* has gone out of balance. Daily sleeping in will make you prone to increasing *kapha* imbalance. Since *kapha* is strong in the morning and evening it is wise to eat lightly at those times. Digestion awakens slowly in the morning, while during the evening the body is slowing down ready for sleep. Overeating at these times overwhelms digestion.

*Pitta* comes in over the midday period, when the sun is high. The fire element is strong in nature at this time, and fire transforms. Our digestive fire is strongest at midday, which is why this is often the traditional time for a big meal. Apart from in very hot climates, where the intensity of the sun's heat weakens people, eating the main meal is best at midday and soothes *pitta*.

From 2pm to 6pm is the day's *vata* time – the time to take it easier. If *vata* is balanced, this will be a good time for mental work. However, if *vata* is out of balance we may start to feel an energy dip or tiredness at this time.

# THE CYCLE OF THE NIGHT

The evening, from 6pm to 10pm, is *kapha* time, a time for slowing down, eating lightly and preparing for sleep. *Pitta* comes up between 10pm and 2am, and now the transformation function of *pitta* is put to the purpose of healing after the day's activities. This is the time to replenish, to restore energies, remove toxins and replace distorted structures in the body. This is what happens when we sleep at this time. People with strong *pitta* may tend to stay up late as they feel *pitta* rising and they come alive with more energy. However, being in bed before 10pm keeps *pitta* better balanced.

Vata comes up between 2am and 6am, and the mind is now active even in sleep, as we dream. This is the time for the mind to renew itself, as the body did in *pitta* time. So the experiences of the day are organized, memories consolidated and the mind refreshed for the next day during this period of restful activity. If you have *vata* out of balance you will find yourself awake at 4am. Then you may not sleep until after 6am, when *kapha* time comes.

# HEALTHY CYCLES

The cycles come and go. As they do so we feel their vary-
ing qualities. If we choose to do the appropriate things to
balance during these changing times we keep well and
happy. If we are ignorant of their effects or choose to do
our own thing regardless, we bear the consequences.

An awareness of this can transform people's lives for
the better. So many people suffer *vata* problems of anxiety, insomnia and aches and pains, but they continue to
disturb vata by rushing, missing lunch and going to bed
late, in a totally unnatural regime for them. Insomnia is
not treated at bedtime – it is treated during the day. If
*vata* is kept balanced between 2pm and 6pm, it will not
be so excited as to wake you between 2am and 6am.

The real secret is to know your own state of *vata*, *pitta*
and *kapha*. For example, your *kapha* may need minding.
This could be either because of a tendency to *kapha*
imbalance or because of a strong *kapha* in your nature. If
so you would need to avoid sleep-ins and overeating at
night and be especially vigilant in winter to take exercise

and the *kapha*-reducing foods. If *pitta* requires balancing, you would focus on a good lunch, a reasonable bedtime and relaxing more in summer. A *vata* nature requires regular routines of bed and mealtimes, with plenty of rest, especially in autumn.

This is not difficult. It may require a change of old habits. But when those old habits don't really suit you, it comes as a relief to stop them. Doing what is best for us feels good, so we like to do it. Returning to the old pattern causes old discomforts to recur. So motivation grows.

A computer comes with vast instruction manuals, but the body is an even more sophisticated machine – and the instruction manual is within the machine itself. It is not difficult for us to recognize what suits us when we are in good health. We feel and function better when we live in tune with our nature. However, when we become ill, we lose this insight and no longer know what we need. Living against our nature causes trouble and disease.

When we are ill, Ayurveda helps us to recognize how to heal. When we are well, it encourages that style of living that constantly rejuvenates.

# YOUR CHALLENGE

To be healthier you need to know what to do. The "knowledge of life", Ayurveda, offers you this insight. You have now read about this knowledge, and for more detailed and precise help you can consult a well-trained Ayurveda practitioner.

Most people will have recognized some basic changes that may improve their health. There might be a few things you know you ought to do. But knowing is not enough. If you are *kapha*, all the wisdom in the world will not improve your health if you continue to overeat and avoid exercise. If you are *vata*, knowledge alone is no use if you overwork and continue an irregular routine. And knowing that you are *pitta* will not help if you take on too much work in too short a time or eat heating foods.

You have to actually make the changes in order to feel the benefits, and making changes can be a challenge. I hope the insights gained from Ayurveda will motivate you to take up this challenge. You can create better health – so now just go and do it!

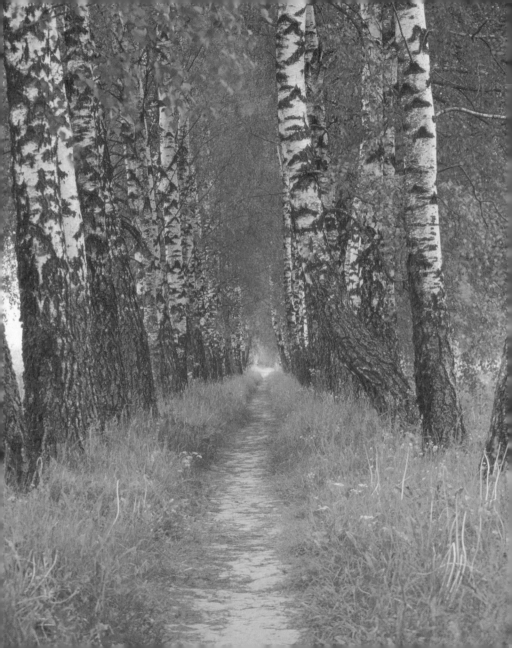

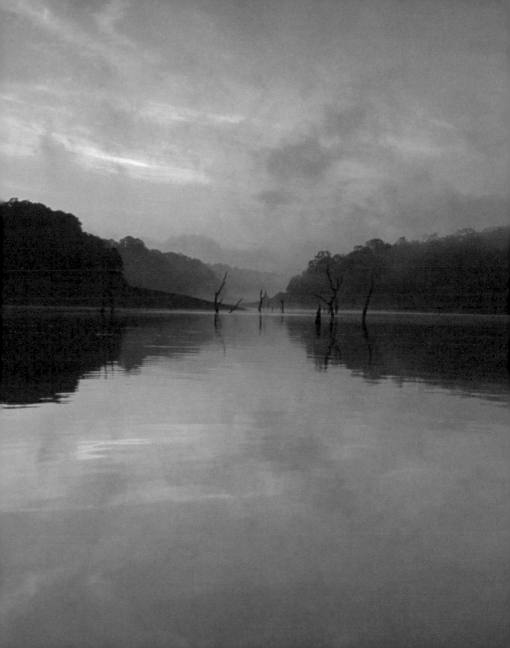

Your treasure house is within;
it contains all you'll ever need.

HUI-HAI

(720–814)

Life is not merely to be alive, but to be well.

MARCUS VALERIUS MARTIAL

(c40–c103CE)

# INDEX

# PICTURE CREDITS / ACKNOWLEDGMENTS

## Picture Credits

The publisher would like to thank the following people and photographic libraries for permission to reproduce their material. Every care has been taken to trace copyright holders. However, if we have omitted anyone we apologize and will, if informed, make corrections in any future edition.

**Page 1** BM/Prod/Getty Images; **2** Dinodia Photo Library; **13** A Green/Zefa /Corbis; **17** G.Kalt/Zefa/ Corbis; **19** P. Dyballa/Zefa/Corbis; **20** Macduff Everton/Corbis; **22** Mehau Kulyk/ Science Photo Library; **25** Laureen March/Corbis; **26** BM/Prod/Getty Images; **31** A. Inden/Zefa/Corbis; **33** A Green/Zefa/Corbis; **37** Trevor Mein/Stone/Getty Images; **38** Corbis; **41** Roland Gerth/Zefa/ Corbis; **43** Sasha/Photonica/Getty Images; **44** Henning Von Holleben/Photonica/Getty Images; **47** Jim Erickson/Corbis; **49** Jonathan Knowles/Photonica/Getty Images; **50** Eric Meola/Image Bank/Getty Images; **53** Steve Cole/Image Bank/Getty Images; **54** Uwe Krejci/Stone/Getty Images; **57** Reg Charity/Corbis; **61** Catherine Karnow/Corbis; **67** LWA-Stephen Welstead/Zefa/Corbis; **71** Jeremy Maude/Digital Vision/Getty Images; **72** Surfpix; **75** John Terence Turner/Taxi/Getty Images; **76** Envision/Corbis; **79** Diana Healey/Botanica/Getty Images; **80** James Day/Photonica/Getty Images; **91** Bruce Burkhardt/Corbis; **92** Laurence Monneret/Stone/Getty Images; **98** Alan.P.Barnes/Taxi/ Getty Images; **103** Altrendo Images/Getty Images; **104** John Henley/Corbis; **107** Cheque/Corbis; **109** Michael Orton/Photographer's Choice/Getty Images; **110** H. Kehrer/Zefa/Corbis; **113** G. Rossenbach/Zefa/Corbis; **114** Craig Tuttle/Corbis; **119** Charles Kreb/Corbis; **123** TETSU/Getty Images; **124** Frans Lanting/Corbis

## Author's Acknowledgments

Maharishi Mahesh Yogi is the greatest scientist in the field of consciousness. He is best known for reviving interest in meditation around the world since introducing Transcendental Meditation in the 1950s. He continues his work in reviving and disseminating all the different sciences from the ancient Vedic tradition, including Ayurveda. For any further information please see www.mapi.com.

Maharishi was my main teacher and he also organized for me to live and study with Dr Subhedar, Dr C.P. Shukla and Dr Hanumanth Rao. Dr Raju over the past two decades has been a wise and compassionate teacher. Many other Ayurvedic practitioners instructed and inspired me and I bow to their wisdom and love.

Many teachers of Transcendental Meditation over the years offered me support in disseminating the wisdom of Ayurveda. Paul and Sarah Matthews are a joy to work with. I thank them all for their help and support.

Grace Cheetham at Duncan Baird Publishers is a tower of strength and initiative, and I thank her and her staff for their kind guidance.

Finally, it is from patients that a doctor learns most. It is in gratitude to them that I have written this book, in the hope of its helping them, and you, to be healthier.